INNER *Focus*
Outer STRENGTH

Using Imagery and Exercise for Strength, Health and Beauty

Eric Franklin

D0746564

Elysian Editions
Princeton Book Company, Publishers

071820045

Please note:
This book will help you become more flexible. It provides information that can help you to help yourself. It does not replace medical advice. When in doubt, experiencing sustained or acute pain, or suffering from illness, you should consult a doctor or other qualified health professional.

Originally published as *Locker sein macht stark*
© 1998 fur die deutsche Ausgabe by Kösel-Verlag GmbH & Co., München

Elysian Editions
Princeton Book Company, Publishers
614 Route 130
Hightstown, NJ 08520

Translated by Frances Shem Barnett and Arja Laubaucher
Illustrated by Sonja Burger and Katharina Hartmann

Design by Mulberry Tree Press and Lisa Denham
Composition by Mulberry Tree Press
Cover design by John McMenamin

Cataloging-in-Publication data
Franklin, Eric N.
[Locker sein macht stark. English]
Inner Focus, Outer Strength: Using Imagery and Exercise for Health, Strength and Beauty / Eric Franklin.
p.: ill. ; cm.
    Includes index and bibliographical references.
    ISBN-10: 0-87127-288-1
    ISBN-13: 978-0-87127-288-1
    1. Fitness. 2. Using imagery. 3. Mind and body.

RA781 .F7313 2006
613.7

Printed in Canada
8   7   6   5   4   3

For my parents,
Joan and Jules Franklin

Contents

Acknowledgements

I thank my family for their patience with "Papa" who has been writing all the time. I thank all the people who inspire me: Bonnie Cohen, André Bernard, Martha Myers, Zvi Gotheiner, Cathy Ward, and many others, including illustrators Sonja Burger and Katharina Hartmann, who have so exquisitely converted my sketches. I also thank my parents who have allowed me to live out my creativity.

Introduction

The marathon runner on the home stretch

Everyone can improve his or her physical performance. Flexibility, economy of movement, a good posture and the use of imagery are important ways to achieve this.

Flexibility and looseness improve strength because of the number of joints and the corresponding muscles that are at our disposal for executing a given movement. Inflexibility leads to the overtaxing of certain joints, while others are harmed by lack of use. A joint that is not used stiffens at an astonishing rate, and the stiffness in each area has to be overcome with additional effort. Energy is then wasted.

Through flexibility, you will not only be stronger in your movements, but these movements will also be more efficient. I will show you how, with minimal effort, you can reach the greatest freedom of movement possible. This alone is not enough, of course; one of the most important goals to be reached is a sense of well-being felt throughout the entire body. When the body feels well, mental achievements of the highest kind are not far away.

Top athletes often speak of feelings of harmony, of experiences of effortless perfection, during their best performances. At the first sign of exhaustion, a marathon runner may imagine a path of clouds under his feet, and a following wind that carries him to the finish line. Helpful winds and the harmonious flow of movement can be part of less spectacular efforts, through imagery. What is the good of all the busyness of daily life if the result is stress, cramps and pain?

Fitness

It's 5:30 P.M. and you have spent the whole day in the office. Now it is time to go to the fitness center to get some exercise, to get on a bike, to have a swim, or to have a run in the fresh air. The muscles are sluggish with disuse, the joints have not been getting enough exercise, the blood is fighting its way through tissue, toxins are stuck in the body.

But liberation approaches. Your training should start with a warm-up, so that the muscles and joints are prepared and do not feel suddenly taken by surprise. The body has to make a complete U-turn: for the whole day, it seemed that physical movement was as extinct as a dinosaur, then suddenly there is a frenzy of movement. The muscles will try to create tonicity as fast as possible, and the production of lubricating synovial fluid may lag behind what is needed for the joints. The lymph system, which has accumulated toxins that can be dealt with only ineffectively because of the lack of movement during the day, may now become overwhelmed. The heart and blood vessels will react to the sudden strain, and the ligaments may suffer if there is a lack of balance.

During the day, the focus was on mental activity. Now it is the body's turn—for an hour, maybe more, usually less. Or none!

The human body is built to move a lot. Human beings are not a sitting, lying, or standing apparatus with a nutshell at the top carrying a computer that needs to be nourished.

After efficient exercise, one feels loose, elastic, aired-out, refreshed and positive. What would it be like to have this feeling throughout the day? Sudden fierce attacks of movement at a specific hour are not necessarily healthy for the body. It is not what you do from time to time for the body, but what you do habitually that is decisive to your fitness. Time spent in the gym or at sports should be a continuation of a day-long awareness of one's body and its fitness.

Mental and physical fitness cannot be separated. The functioning of our mental faculties is based on our hereditary disposition and the sum of all our physical experiences. Without the correct functioning of sensory perception, the brain doesn't have meaningful input. Similarly, important information for the brain comes from movement, posture and your sense of balance.

Fitness is also a matter of attitude and is not only based on physical exercise. Good exercises regularly done are a good beginning, but not the end, of getting and staying fit. Fitness training should not be reduced to being seen as a pill to be taken in response to unhealthy behavior. To be really fit, I think that the feeling of *joy in movement* is necessary.

Motivation for movement

We go to a gym or find another training program. This certainly is a great start, but what is the motivation for going to the gym? The desire to tone the body and have a firm bottom? The fear of becoming ill? The feeling of well-being just after training? The key factor of fitness training is not *what* but *how*. Any training carried out with a bit of humor, elasticity and awareness will do something for one's health. Training is no guarantee for improvement in flexibility or for the loosening of tension. Tense exercising will promote a tense posture and breathing. Again and again I have observed that even people who breathe in a relaxed manner put their most important breathing muscle, the diaphragm, under pressure. The execution of movements should be done with as much economy as possible.

Economy of movement without mental *presence* is impossible. Presence during training happens effortlessly if one delights in movement. Whatever is done with presence will succeed better, whether baking a cake or making a properly-executed knee bend.

I have written this book to help you find something entirely revolutionary: delight in moving, so that the fitness program that you are doing, or considering doing, will benefit both your body and mind to the maximum.

There is nothing more tiring than having to do something in which you are not interested. What happened to the spontaneous joy of movement that we had as children? Have we been told too often that sitting still is good, while romping around wildly is bad?

Also, one cannot put too much emphasis on the fact that beauty and health come from within. A superficial fitness and health training will let you down sooner or later. The inner approach is as important as the outer activity. Fitness, which should be a life-long goal, builds on inner strength. This book is about developing inner strength, health and beauty.

Stress

Tension, back pain and stress will not suddenly appear one day. I maintain that most of these problems are created over time by our behavior. Stress is the unconscious (or learned) decision to react to certain events with too much physical or mental tension. Most situations that cause stress in daily life don't demand such a strong reaction and could be faced with more ease. In reality we meet with our own reactions and not with unalterable facts (unless a Bengal tiger crosses our way). For many, stress is a kind of *fata morgana*, the illusion that more is achieved if one surrounds oneself with a hectic atmosphere; that those who work in a relaxed and loose way are not giving their utmost. Exhaustion and good work performance do not belong together! The opposite is true:

those who perform in a relaxed way will perform with more precision and creativity and will make fewer mistakes.

The upshot is that stress is a habit and therefore can be given up without achieving less. On the contrary, without stress one will achieve more and for more years to come!

The experience journal

Before starting with the actual exercise part of this book, I would like to suggest that readers note experiences they have while exercising. Drawings and sketches should be allowed to arise from within us without expectation or perfection. I have found that registering an experience helps progress tremendously. This is how new insight and each new *body feeling* will stay more *present* and make up the elements for the next experience to anchor changes in the consciousness of the self.

Here is an example: imagine that your shoulders are melting like vanilla ice cream in the sun. Imagine that the shoulders glide down the side of the body. The neck muscles become long and relaxed, the neck becomes free and the head floats like a balloon on top of the spine. You can actually feel a certain relaxation from this imagery. Make notes of the experience. Then, when you don't think about it for a while, suddenly—perhaps at work or on your way home—the image pops up in your mind: "Yes—my shoulders are really melting like vanilla ice, now I've got it again." Maybe there is a new element in this second experience: "I can feel that my spine is somehow longer." At home you write down this new experience and in this way your progress speeds up enormously. You start to understand how the body functions. It seems that your spine can get longer just by letting go of the shoulders.

It is exciting and instructive to read through your journal after a few months and see how your body feeling has changed in the course of time. We see that children draw and color a lot and are thus working through their experiences in their daily lives. Unfortunately, many adults believe that they can't draw—instead of just trying it out.

Start right now with a drawing of yourself. Try to draw yourself from the front and the side. Close your eyes and picture an image of your shape. Draw this image. Each month, repeat this exercise. You will discover amazing differences in your drawings. The body gives us the chance to have boundless experiences and find out fundamental things about ourselves and the world. This book attempts to help you to walk that path.

1 Our Body Helps Us Think

Many people fill a good part of their daily thoughts with unpleasant scenarios as reflected in the booming health insurance business. Instead of paying to insure ourselves against illness, we should focus on our own built-in insurance: our bodies. I am convinced that positive awareness of the body is good for our health. Insuring ourselves means being aware of the inevitable decline of the body. Do we place more trust in an insurance policy than in the self-healing power of our body? It seems that way. To sit quietly, to focus on breathing and visualize that at each moment three thousand million blood corpuscles are busy transporting oxygen to the cells of our body does the body a wealth of good; we are giving it positive attention. I maintain that each cell in the body can "feel," if we just have trust in our bodies. Each living cell in our body has the possibility to communicate; everything going on in the body can be felt. We should be wary of the widespread belief that we are not supposed to feel something if it isn't scientifically proven.

Work and the body

Wouldn't it be great if your work, whatever it might be, is good for your body? Do you believe that work tires out your body? Imagine a life in which each and every movement is constructive and refreshing; where each time you move it feels pleasant and agreeable, and you look forward to each movement because you know you are doing something good for your body. Does this sound to you like excessive positive thinking? It is a fact that every move we make gives us a kind of inner massage. Organs, muscles, bones and connective tissues glide over each other, nestle into each other, twist and turn in an inner dance, and all this enables our inherent flexibility. Without this inner flexibility, our movements would be stiff and clumsy.

Flexibility comes not only from stretching our muscles. We wouldn't even be able to bend forward if our inner organs didn't cooperate. The lungs, for example, are separated into lobes. Three are found on the right, and two on the left: there are just two on the left to accommodate the heart. If you bend forward, these lobes slide like soap sponges over each other and allow a change in the shape of the thorax. If lungs were inflexible, your thorax would be as stiff as a block of wood. Lack of movement stiffens not only the muscles and joints, but also the organs and all other structures in the body. They start to literally stick to each other, and the ability to glide decreases. The consequences are not only muscle cramps, but also indigestion and circulation disorders. Movement becomes more and more difficult, and in the end many people experience movement as exhausting and unpleasant.

Our goal should therefore be to improve the joy of movement and the flexibility of the whole body, not only of the muscles and joints. In this context, I will elaborate on a few topics that are connected to our attitudes to movement in general.

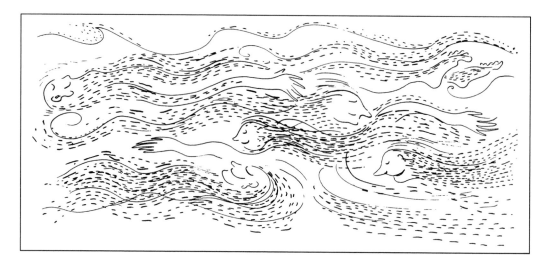

Movement as inner massage

Imagine that every movement we make massages us inside. Visualize the many layers and membranes in our body: the skin, the muscles with their sheaths of connective tissue, the bones and their *periosteum* (the protective membrane of connective tissue covering them), and the organs with their coverings (*peritoneum* and *pulmonary pleura*). These can move, glide and shift around each other. Imagine that this inner gliding is a pleasant massage for the tissues. Each movement leads to a sense of well-being.

How we talk about the body

Again and again I notice that people usually have something negative to say about their bodies: "Today my lower back hurts, and the pain in my knee won't go away." On the other hand, people find it strange if one is too positive about one's body: "Today my body feels really lively, every tendon and muscle feels elastic, my joints are supple and delight in movement!" If these statements apply to you, I congratulate you. Most people react to such statements by smiling slightly— anyone who speaks that way is weird and must have a screw loose!

Let me emphasize that I am not suggesting we ignore our physical ailments. Getting medical treatment in some cases is essential. I want to emphasize, rather, that there exists a connection between our physical health and those of our body's experiences we choose to focus on. If we dwell on negative experiences alone, these will be in the forefront of our minds and will thus be encouraged. But if we also focus on positive experiences, these will be reinforced, and any negative feelings will diminish. It's like a talent show: instead of just criticizing poor performances, let us enjoy exciting discoveries.

Hope is medicine. To impress on the body that its state is hopeless will deprive it of hope and healing. This concept isn't necessarily an unrealistic fantasy. You accept the reality, assess the situation realistically, and do your best to improve the situation through your own thoughts and actions. Even for someone in a poor physical state, it is possible to find a joint or muscle that moves smoothly and with pleasure. From this simple premise, a new "body feeling" can be created, as the joy of movement is contagious.

Tales of the body

What kind of sensations do you have in your body in this instant? Think about what you would tell a good friend about your body. Ask yourself the following questions:

1. Where do I feel pressure or pain?

2. Which parts of my body don't feel good?

3. Is there a spot that feels good?

4. Is there a spot that feels great?

5. Can you describe this great feeling in more detail?

6. What happens if a good spot encounters a not-so-good spot? Can that spot learn something from the good one?

Pleasure comes to the rescue

I feel pressure in my lower back on the right side. There seems to be a tense muscle there. When I straighten my back, I feel a certain pain. My breathing in the front part of my thorax feels pleasant, light and soft, like a silk cushion filled with downy feathers. I try to feel both places at the same time: the pleasant, light feeling, and the tense one. Mentally I confront them with each other. I realize that the light, soft cushion inspires the tense muscle. It still hurts a little, but it is already a lot softer. I keep focusing on the lightness and the...where has the tense spot vanished to?

I am not saying that your experience will always be as smooth as the one described above, but keep an open mind. Write down your thoughts in your journal (see Introduction) and repeat this exercise as often as you wish. You can also put to good use unexpected idle moments waiting for a train, a bus, or at a red light.

Wishes for the body

Open a new page in your journal and write the following: "Wishes for my body." Below this write down all the things you wish for your body. Formulate your wishes positively:

1. Loose shoulders

2. Flexible back

3. Deep breathing

4. Lively feet

5. ... and what other wishes you may have.

The problem obsession

Changing our attitude toward our body is an essential step toward healing a physical problem. For many people who receive medical treatment, the problem will disappear for a short while, if at all. If I ask a group of physiotherapists during one of my courses if they know clients with a "problem obsession," I see a lot of nodding heads. Or to put it another way, when the patient's knee is healed, it is the foot's turn next month, and then the back, and so on. I believe that we have to make a basic shift in our thinking if we really want to free ourselves from the "problem obsession."

First, one has to find trust in the self-healing capabilities of the body and re-discover that movement is fun. The body is capable of mobilizing unbelievable powers but only if we support it with a positive attitude. We have to learn to discover the joy in our body again—in fact, right down to our cells. Loose, relaxed movement is the laughter of the body.

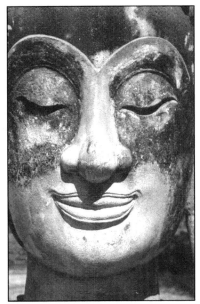

I don't claim that this is easy. After all, many people have experienced the opposite in a most painful way. Moving hurts, and a long and painful battle with pain isn't exactly motivating. The first step is to think about what positive things the pain or the problem may have brought you. Even though everyone has different experiences with physical problems, I believe that an enormous ability for concentration can result from them; the scattered mind is focused through the pain on one goal: "What do I have to do to get well?" People are guided to wholly different paths in their lives through illness or pain. We may also be led to questioning our behavior, or the sense of our actions. New goals are set, and the unimportant is separated from the important. We feel that nobody can know our body as intimately as we can. And the more we are interested in the experience of our body, the more success we will have with and through it.

The cells laugh

Imagine that each of your cells has a face (the photo shows the inner smile of the Buddha). What does this look like? Does it laugh or cry? Is it grumpy and suspicious or happy and light? Do all cells in the body have the same face? Are there cells in your body that are able to laugh out loud? Does an enormous choir of laughing, cheering and singing cells develop? Draw your experiences in your diary.

Mental recycling

The recycling of material is not the only way to recycle; we can also recycle mentally. Suppose that instead of filling ourselves with benevolent and constructive thoughts, we load ourselves with mental garbage. Luckily, as well as recycling kitchen garbage, we can also recycle our mental orientation. One has to find a way to transform the large and small piles of doubt, anger, fear, envy and jealousy that accumulate during the day, as these feelings harm us most. Every time we get angry with someone, our cells wince and charge themselves with unnecessary tension. We forget that each mental vibration we send out also touches us (as it is created by us), before it can be targeted at somebody else. Fortunately we have the "negativity-absorber."

The negativity-absorber

This exercise is especially recommended before going to sleep, to free oneself of unnecessary burdens. It often makes sleep deeper and more restful.

Sit or lie down comfortably and imagine that there is a "negative-absorber" at your disposal. This negativity-absorber has the ability to suck up negative thoughts like a vacuum cleaner, and transform them into a harmless "thought-puree." This thought-puree then becomes the source of benevolent and constructive thoughts, symbolized by flowers. The negative thoughts leave the body as a kind of soot or grey-black smoke or in any way you'd like to visualize them. The absorber can also concentrate on particular regions of the body, but in general it will need to work on the whole body. The negativity-absorber starts at your feet, picks up all the negative soot and smoke, and then continues on to the knees and the pelvis, pulling all negativity from the body. It floats slowly up the body to the top of your head. Sooty, sticky and blocked snatches of thought—everything negative that we have burdened ourselves with—are all sucked up indiscriminately. Perhaps the negativity-absorber will linger over a certain spot in order to do more in-depth work. Visualize the soot coming out of every body part, every cell. All the negativity-dust is buried. Out of this ground grow beautiful flowers with smiling faces, radiating joy.

Movement as delight

Life is movement. Why not enjoy it? No one will prevent you from moving except yourself. Even if you were only able to move your little finger, it would still be worthwhile to try and find enjoyment in that. Ask yourself, "Is there any movement I would like to do right now? Is there any stretching, yawning or sighing that would make me feel better?" Make a few pleasurable movements, like a cat stretching after a little nap.

Waking up the senses

For this exercise you will need a partner who will lead you around a room, ideally a room full of interesting objects. Close your eyes or wrap a blindfold around them. In this exercise, you should feel your way around with your hands, without looking. Your partner leads you to different objects in the room. Feel them with your fingers and try to guess what the objects are. After five or ten minutes, open your eyes and see how your body feels. By using your senses so intensely, you may have found a new sense of your body.

Diversity of movement

Movement exercises that focus on discovering pleasure in the body freshen and strengthen more than purely goal-oriented exercises. No other animal is able to make so many different kinds of movements: we can crawl like a crocodile, but a crocodile cannot walk like a human.

The spontaneous need for movement can be especially observed in small children playing, scuffling and tussling. Young animals even put themselves in danger just to get the chance to play, tease and romp around. In many situations, such spontaneity does not fit in the adult world. Our surroundings are sometimes in such a way that they prevent spontaneity and creativity.

Back experience

My back felt tense, so I wanted to do a relaxation exercise. As I was lying down on the ground in preparation, my children jumped on me and we started a playful tussle that lasted about ten minutes. Afterwards I was surprised to find that my back was wonderfully relaxed. I had experienced for myself the therapeutic effect of a good tussle. Children move with great joy and astonishing diversity until they learn that good behavior is somehow connected with less movement. As a consequence, hundreds of joints thirst every day to show off their tricks, but we hardly give them a chance to do so.

Can you remember yourself as a child scuffling and tussling as you played with your siblings and friends? Try it out today—one is never too old for it. Tussle with your children or "fight" with a big cushion. You will notice that not only does your respiratory rate increase, but your mood also lifts.

The voice

What is true of the joints is also true of the voice. Making noises, calling, crying, squealing, yelling—children do them often and like to do them, as they know intuitively how important the voice is for the development of the breathing organs and the activation of the locomotor system. I was once with a colleague on the train to a workshop in Munich, when we suddenly laughed aloud after about two hours of the journey. The reaction was immediate: there came sharp "pssst!" from the neighboring compartment. We cringed, startled. Obviously laughter was out of place around here. The reaction of the body to laughing out loud points to the connection between voice and body.

Voice and movement

1. Press your lips together, stretch your arms upwards and lower them again.

2. Relax your lips by exhaling through them, vibrating while making a "prrrrr" sound.

3. Breathe out with an "Aah" sound while lifting and lowering your arms.

4. Which one is easier? When is there more tension in the shoulders?

Spontaneity

Humans move spontaneously from the fetal stage. Nevertheless, I have noticed in my courses that people are puzzled if faced with the task of moving according to their feelings, without any instructions. We have forgotten what it means to be spontaneous and to feel which movements our body likes making. As adults, our movements tend to serve a purpose: walking through the grocery store, using a computer, cooking soup, brushing teeth—our movements usually have a purpose. Even in the gym, our movements serve a purpose: strengthening certain muscles, exercising particular joints, supplying tissues with blood. It is interesting that before birth, the first senses to come into action are hearing and balance. Our first experiences in the womb are of twisting and turning, of paddling and pushing, as every expectant mother knows well.

After birth, the movement of babies and infants is characterized by delight and joy and is essential for the development of the brain. Yet these primeval exercises are seldom carried on into adulthood. Slowly the child learns that there are certain given sets of important movements which one is supposed to learn. At first, he or she goes about this task with much joy, but as prescribed movements are learned, the joy begins to diminish, and the spontaneous delight of movement is lost.

In the following exercise, you will rediscover the relaxing and restful effect of spontaneous movement. At first this may seem difficult without a model for these movements, but given time you will never want to give up spontaneous movement again.

The spontaneous desire to move

This exercise should be done in pairs (and is especially suitable for the outdoors):

Person A should move however he or she wishes. Person B should support the movements of his or her partner with the hands, for example with a light tapping on the back. Person A should give feedback to Person B as to whether the tapping is pleasant, or whether it should be lighter or harder, for example. A should now close his or her eyes for the rest of the exercise. After a few minutes, B should withdraw so that A moves alone. B should watch A so that he or she doesn't bump into things. The exercise should last at least ten minutes, but could be longer. After B has told A that the time is up, A should rest with his or her eyes closed, then slowly open them. A should look around, noting that things may look a bit different now. Before A and B change roles, they can give each other feedback or write something about their experience. Then the mover and the helper change roles.

Touch

I think that human touch plays an important role in fitness and health. In general, there should be more touching, not only for healing illnesses, or comforting children and older people, but also in daily life. From my school days, I clearly remember a psychological experiment described in a textbook. Researchers had shown that a baby chimpanzee preferred a wire frame "mother" with a soft covering, without food, to a a wire frame with food but without a soft cover. The baby animal was clutching at the cover and snuggling up to it. Of course, I felt very sorry for it and hoped that it would soon be reunited with its real mother. Just like scuffling and tussling, warmth and security, cuddling and snuggling, touching and being touched are needs that all animals (especially mammals) have in common with humans.

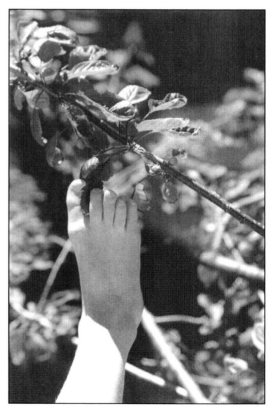

The skin is an important organ, a protective covering weighing approximately thirteen pounds. It breathes, secretes and absorbs, provides warmth and shelter, and gives us information about our environment. The latest research shows that the importance of touch is even greater than originally assumed: without the opportunity to play, and without enough physical contact through touching, the brain cannot develop properly. Children who lack being touched and play time have less brain matter. Additionally, we know how important touch is for premature babies: they gain weight much faster if they are touched regularly. But with adults, too, touching stimulates the development of the brain, which never ceases. As long as we are alive, we can create new connections between neurons. The more trained we are at using touch, the more we can achieve with this skill. I believe that one's state of being is an integral part of this training. If you are comfortable in your own body, you will be able to use touch in a pleasant way. If tired or tense, you will transfer this feeling to another person.

As is to be expected, concentration and imagery play an important role in touch: they guide our hands. If we think of our breathing as soft, free and relaxed, and then touch somebody, this will help to transfer our feeling of relaxation. The livelier our imagery, the greater is our touching potential. For example, heart surgeon Mehmet Oz, of Columbia Presbyterian Hospital in New York, has a Therapeutic Touch specialist to assist him during surgery. He knows from experience that with therapeutic touch, pain after surgery is reduced, and blood pressure and heart rates are lowered.

Touch meditation

Touch the arm of a partner with your hands. Maybe you can feel some warmth; perhaps you can also feel something else–allow yourself to be surprised. Wait patiently and observe with your sense of touch what is going on under your hands. Imagine that this is a kind of meditation meant to empty the head of thoughts and to help you simply feel. Know that your very awareness, your presence, and the meeting of two people through touch, can have an effect. Continue touching: it represents your simply "being here." After five to ten minutes, take your hands away. Your partner should compare the feeling in each arm. Talk to each other about what you experienced.

2 Flexibility

Flexibility and body awareness

Flexibility is attained not just by the exercises suggested here but also through a refining of body awareness. Some people who are very flexible in certain joints can't transfer this *partial* flexibility to an *overall* flexibility. Then again, there are those who have only limited flexibility in their joints but look very flexible when moving. Humans are not machines, and the mobility of the joints is not the sole deciding factor in general flexibility. So how can we learn to make the most of our flexibility? By feeling where we are already flexible! I emphasize that in this case *feeling* should not be confused with *knowing*. We can know, for example, that the foot has many joints without actually feeling them—and this will hardly contribute to our flexibility. The more precisely we can feel where movement in the body can happen, the bigger the potential for flexibility—just as a complete and exact sense of the body enables more precise movement. In order to direct a movement, there are precise maps and routes at the disposal of the brain. If you move your arm and have difficulty feeling the shoulder joint, you will not be as flexible as someone who can feel that the movement of the arm is enabled through the shoulder blade gliding on the thorax. Those who know how to support and refine movement spare their joints, as no single joint has to take care of the movement alone.

Presence in moving

The more consciously *present* you are during a movement, the more flexibility is at your disposal. If you follow a change of body position with the inner eye, you have more ability to steer the movement precisely. The conscious observing of events in the joints during exercising improves flexibility, since the nervous system attains a refined control of movement through this conscious support. This saves you a great deal of time in the end, because the newly found flexibility anchors into the brain and becomes a permanent state. Now the brain will be able to give the shoulders and arms more detailed movement orders: when we put the telephone to our ear, our shoulders and neck are relaxed and free of tension. It is clear to our nervous system which muscles and joints should be used, and which ones should not. Without this improved awareness, we will become repeatedly tense and cramped, regardless of any relaxation exercises. Those who are only occasionally present in their bodies will miss many opportunities for adjusting and refining movement. Being present in the body is effortless, can have a positive influence on hormonal balance, and leads to a comfortable state of the body comparable to that known to many dancers. Being "physically awake" during movement leads to an increased secretion of endorphins, the endogenous painkiller, and conscious movement feels exceedingly good. On the other hand, mental absence during movement will tend to render exercise more strenuous and exhausting.

Swinging the arm

1. Continuously swing your right arm forward and backward during this exercise. Imagine first that your arm swings from the shoulder joint; the movement of the arm is triggered by the shoulder joint.

2. Now imagine that the swing of the arm is also supported by the movements of the shoulder blade and the collarbone. The shoulder blade glides in a relaxed fashion on the thorax.

3. Imagine that the swing of the arm is also achieved by the elastic movement of the thorax. The thorax helps to make the swing of the arm possible.

4. Imagine that the swing of the arm is also supported by the gliding of the lungs in the thorax. The lungs are like sponges that encourage the thorax from within toward an even more complete movement. Allow your breathing to be very relaxed.

5. Imagine now that the swing of the arm is also made possible by the spine. The spine helps to swing the arm.

6. Let the swinging of the arm come to an end and compare the looseness of the right and the left shoulders. Stretch the arms forward and compare the length of the arms.

7. Repeat the same exercise on the left side of the body.

Where is flexibility located?

A joint is, simply put, a space between two bones. This space is filled with a slippery liquid called *synovia* which allows completely smooth gliding of the two cartilage-covered bones. There are hundreds of joints in the body that are filled with this synovial fluid. Flexibility in the joints means that the two facing joint surfaces are able to glide in opposite directions from each other. Inflexibility in a joint means that the same points of the joint surfaces are always opposite each other. This is a disadvantage for the cartilage that depends on a good distribution of the synovial fluid, This distribution is achieved by the gliding movement massaging it into the cartilage. If there is a lack of synovial fluid, the cartilage is not nourished sufficiently and starts to degenerate. In the worst case, osteoarthritis can develop. Furthermore, the neighboring joints have to compensate, often in unfavorable circumstances. So, a joint that hurts often hasn't caused the problem itself.

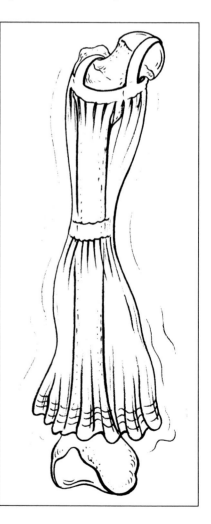

All this may sound familiar. However, we are less aware of our organs. Organs are not as hard as bones and cartilage, but are also surrounded by fluid, and can glide over each other. Incidentally, this is also true for many tissues in the body; they are able to shift over each other like bones in a joint. Even single cells can move. Cells are surrounded by fluid that nourishes them, and like joint surfaces, single cells can glide around each other.

Flexibility in our whole body

1. Move with the following questions in mind: "Where am I flexible? Where does flexibility reside in my body?" Feel how countless joint surfaces in the body move smoothly over each

other: the joints of the hip, the knee, the many joints of the feet and hands, the joints of the spine, the shoulders, the elbows and the jaw. The hundreds of joints in our body are moved effortlessly with the help of synovial fluid.

2. There is flexibility of the organs. Imagine that the lungs and the heart are moving flexibly against each other. Imagine that the stomach, the liver, and the intestines are likewise moving flexibly around each other.

3. There is flexibility of the muscles. Visualize the single muscle fibers moving against one another, the bellies of the muscles sliding and gliding over each other.

4. There is flexibility of the muscles and the bones. Visualize the muscles freeing themselves from the bones. Imagine the muscles swinging like a loose summer dress around the bones. It is almost as if the bones were able to move within the muscles, just as our arms are able to move around in loose shirtsleeves.

5. There is flexibility between the organs and the bones. The lungs and the heart are not stuck in the thorax but are able to move within it. The intra-abdominal organs are not stuck to the spine, but have a certain freedom of movement.

Alternatives to stretching

For those who don't know much about stretching, a muscle is brought to its current maximum length and then you try to stretch it a little over its "natural" length. If you pay attention to relaxed breathing and correct posture during stretching, you can have considerable success. Nevertheless, it is true that this philosophy of "going further than you want to" entails a certain amount of stress on the muscle. This can even result in muscular injury, and I have often been asked for advice regarding painfully overstretched muscles.

Actually, there are very effective alternatives to stretching that can bring relief for those with flexibility problems. Muscle stretching is, in many ways, counter-effective. People have shortened muscles because they have a rigid image of their body; they move with too much tension and have bad posture. Forced lengthening of the muscles will only reduce movement tension temporarily. Rigid mental and movement habits will create rigid muscles, while flexible thinking and movement habits will create loose muscles. To start, imagine that your joints are supported by soft clouds (see illustration)

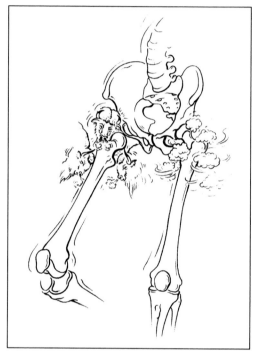

Flexible and flowing muscle movement should not be confused with slackness. On the contrary, there is much strength in flowing movement as any Tai Chi master, and all of us who have been swept off our feet by a wave at the beach, would agree!

I do not advocate that you eliminate stretching. I do suggest that it needs to be combined with a change in mental attitude towards your body and movement if it is to attain permanent results. Even if a muscle is stretched successfully to a certain length, it does not necessarily mean that it will actively reach this newly-gained length. In order to make use of the increased length, sufficient strength and coordination are needed.

When exercising, move the muscle flowingly and consciously into a lengthening position. The muscle needs to learn not only the act of lengthening, but also how to remain there. We will examine this principle more closely in the section entitled "The liberated back" (see page 61). In other words, the muscle needs to get to know the road toward the lengthening, not just the end state.

A further problem with stretching is that often only those muscles that are already sufficiently long get stretched, while not very much happens in other areas. Visualize a rope with knots, the knots representing the tight areas of the muscle. Pull on both ends, and the knots will become even tighter, while the rest of the rope is stretched. Also, if we manage to feel the flexibility and gliding action of a joint, the muscles will adapt to this "joint experience." However, a stretched muscle will not really enable increased control of movement, but only a short-term ability of the joint to stretch. Improvement of the joint experience is crucial for an actively useful flexibility. If we manage to combine an improvement in flexibility with an enhanced movement control, then we gain two advantages: we have attained a lengthening of the muscle without stress on the muscle fibers, and we have also optimized movement control.

One of the signs of movement control is looking at our posture. Our flexibility is only as good as our posture permits. In the case of bad posture, the body's muscles maintain an unbalanced structure and are not available for movement; thus we become less flexible. As soon as posture improves, flexibility increases.

Experience the relationship between posture and flexibility

In your best standing posture, lift your arms overhead, and then lower them again. Notice how flexible your shoulders feel. Now lift and lower your right knee and notice how flexible your hip joint feels. Now slouch your upper body, with head forward and shoulders rounded. Again, lift your arms and notice how flexible the shoulders feel. Perform the knee lift again and sense the flexibility of your hips. Both shoulder and hip flexibility will be reduced in the slouched posture. Repeat the movement in your best upright posture and you will regain the ease and range of motion in your hips and shoulders.

In flow lies strength

Everybody knows how relaxing a hot bath can be. Children love water and splash around in it with an exuberant zest for life. Do you remember when you splashed about in this element, free of gravity? The qualities of water are very relevant for our flexibility: flowing, connecting, changing, expanding, permeating, supporting. Water surrounds us in many variations: fog or clouds that snuggle up to a hill; plump dewdrops that cling to a blade of grass; a wave that continuously splashes against a limestone cliff; a spring that brings clear water from the depths of the earth. Luckily our bodies consist chiefly of water; we carry the qualities of water within us.

Even the form of our body can remind us of water. Bones, under closer scrutiny, look as if they are snapshots of a river, while other places in the body remind us of eddies. If we look at water moving around stones, we discover waves, loops, spirals, and circles. All this can also be found in the human body, which one could say is flow brought into form. One of the goals of flexibility training is to feel the movement that has created this form. If we experience our body as just a fixed form, then we will have a tendency not only toward physical but also mental stagnation. Can we once again feel the movement that lives inside our form? Can we open up new territories to flowing movement?

Remembering the flow

Imagine that you are a stream of water brought into form. Everything we are now, our bones, muscles, every cell, even our thoughts, were once flowing easily. We have emerged from the ocean, from the waves, from the ebb and surge of the tides. Deep inside our being we feel the awakening of the genetic memory of the all-creating flow; we feel the movement of the waves of the primeval ocean.

The living marrow

The innermost part of our bones is the *marrow*. The marrow contains stem cells that produce both the white cells of the immune system and the oxygen-transporting red blood cells. New blood cells are continuously produced at a staggering rate. A million of them are born every second. Count to ten and you have just produced ten million new cells. We are productive at every moment, cellularly speaking, even when we are dozing in the sun.

The marrow is the most liquid part of our bones. To improve the flexibility of your joints, it is very helpful if you visualize the bones as being elastic with a soft center, not as rigid supporting pillars. This image may also help people with osteoporosis and osteoarthritis who do not always experience regenerating life in their bones.

Once, before falling asleep, I had a very strong sensation of feeling the red marrow in my bones, the flexible and liquid center of the entire pelvic region. The next day I woke up with springy, loose and smooth hip joints. I felt as if I were floating. It was also much easier than usual to climb the stairs. I had discovered the liquid in my bones.

The living bone

1. Dive mentally into the center of your bones, the marrow. (The accompanying illustration shows the *trabecular* meshwork, the inner part of the bone.)

2. Feel the powerful center of the bones alive and full of energy.

3. Know that thousands of new cells are being produced here every second, carrying oxygen throughout the body, and bringing new strength to our immune system.

4. Imagine that the marrow can communicate with the whole body.

5. Now go to the peripheral part of the bone, the compact bone. There is a lot going on here as well. With our inner eye we can see the constant rebuilding of our bones and a state of balance.

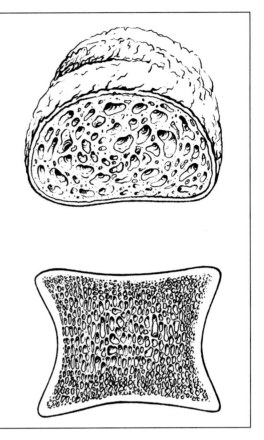

6. Finally, focus your attention on the thin skin around the bone: the periosteum. It is moist and smooth, and nourishes the bone; our muscles can glide effortlessly on this surface, and no muscle will stick to the bone.

7. Move your arms and legs, and finally the whole body, and feel that each movement is also moving the marrow.

8. Rest comfortably with the knowledge that in the very inside of the bones all is well.

Flexibility is contagious

If we manage to become more flexible in one part of the body, then we can feel it right away in other parts as well. There are, however, a few key areas that are crucial to the overall flexibility of the whole body: the feet and the diaphragm.

Massaging the feet

Massage your feet once a day. If you do this in the morning, you will prepare your feet for a buoyant, relaxed day. If you do it in the evening then you will banish the tension of the day from your feet, providing yourself with a deep and restful sleep. You can use massage oil, like arnica or rose oil, or massage your feet in a warm footbath or in your regular bath. You are not primarily concerned with the stimulation of the reflex zones, but with the flexibility of

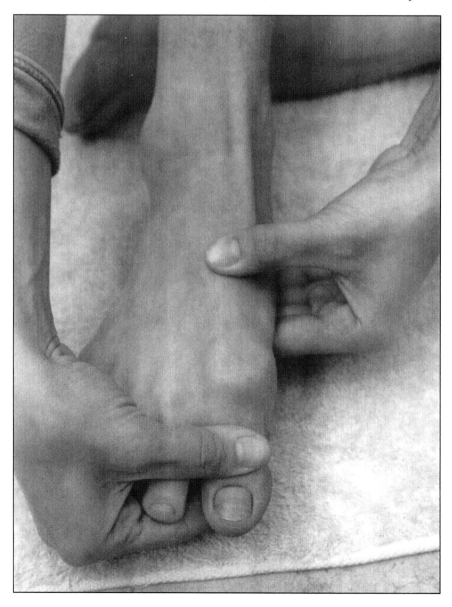

the feet. More flexibility in the feet will promote more flexibility in the entire body and deeper breathing. Make note of the following points as you massage:

1. Relax. Breathe calmly and quietly.

2. Allow your shoulders to stay loose, and don't exert yourself.

3. Draw out the toes as if they were made of chewing gum.

4. The toes are made of three bones, except for the big toe, which has only two bones. There are three joints to consider: a joint at the base of the toe and two more peripheral joints (except in the big toe, which only has one peripheral joint).

5. Visualize the toes starting a bit further back in the foot than they appear. The base joints of the toes are actually to be found further back than the skin indentations between the toes might suggest. When we bend the toes, we can see the protrusion of the base joints on top of the foot (see illustration).

6. Bend and stretch the toes using all the joints of the toes, if you can.

7. Try to loosen the muscles between the bones of the feet. Imagine those muscles becoming downy and soft. Hold your foot with both hands and try to move the bones of the mid-foot (metatarsals) against each other as if you were kneading bread.

8. Knead the heel and rub around both ankles with the fingers in a circular fashion. Flexibility of the ankle is crucial in order to bend and stretch the foot.

9. The sole of the foot has many ligaments and layers of muscle. These may become strained by walking on hard, flat surfaces. Rub your sole so that it becomes soft and smooth.

10. Before massaging the other foot, you should stand up (unless you are in the bathtub, in which case you should stretch yourself out) and compare your two feet. How does the massaged foot feel compared to the other? Try to describe for yourself the difference between them. Perhaps the whole side of the body of the massaged foot feels differently. How do the hip, the back, and the shoulders feel on the massaged side?

3 The Power of Imagery

Sometimes I tell my course participants that I am able to influence their glands without touching them or giving them medicine. There are "Ahs" and "Ohs" as they wait with a certain amount of suspense for the exercise. If you continue to read, your gland system, also, will be influenced with the help of imagery—but have no fear, the exercise can only do you good. It demonstrates the power of imagery on every part of the body, even on every cell: imagine you have a slice of lemon in your mouth. Bite carefully into this slice of lemon and taste and smell the sour flavor. Feel how the sections of lemon burst between your teeth. I am not even able to write this without my saliva starting to flow! The image affects the body immediately and directly.

But why should this exercise be of any use, apart from stimulating the digestion? Chinese medicine tells us that all bodily fluids are connected. If the saliva flows, the fluid distribution in the entire body is improved. Imagine having "saliva glands" around your joints. In this way imagery may even help to ameliorate osteoarthritis. Does this all seem too simplistic? I thought the same way when I started working with imagery for pain in my back, feet and knees many years ago. Now I want to laugh and cry when someone tells me that imagery cannot work in this way. I laugh because it works, in fact, so well, and cry because the person is robbing himself or herself of a great opportunity.

Imagery is deceptively simple and effective, but it has to be trained like a muscle to become effective. There must be strength behind the image. I compare it to language classes: nobody expects to read a Russian newspaper after two lessons in a Russian language. To be really useful, imagery has to be used in daily life again and again, like a language. Many of you are inherently talented at using imagery, and results come fast. Recently there has been much research confirming that imagery is very effective in healing the body, helping athletes win competitions, lifting one's mood, and achieving one's goals. (See Appendix for references.)

A flight to Chicago

I was once on a flight from Zurich to Chicago, in the days when smoking was still allowed on airplanes. As only a thin curtain separated smokers from non-smokers, the smoke easily came into the non-smokers' section. This caused my sinuses to flare up in pain. The air felt as dry and hot as if I were crossing an African desert. I reached for my sinus medication, but, alas, I found I had left it at home. As I was preparing myself for some painful hours to Chicago, I remembered that I was supposed to be a specialist in imagery. If I imagined letting the medicinal drops trickle on my tongue, could it be effective? Would my brain activate my inner medicine chest and reduce my pain? No sooner did I have this thought than it was done. Ten drops of imagery medicine trickled onto my tongue. The result was astonishing: my imaginary drops worked better than my real ones! The headache was gone immediately. The power of imagery allowed me to travel to Chicago without pain.

The soft and relaxed neck

There are certain conditions needed for imagery to work reliably. An important element is the kinesthetic sense, the experience felt in the body. If I hadn't felt the imaginary drops on my tongue as if they were actually there, I would have landed in Chicago with a throbbing head. Kinesthetic images are perceived in the body as if they were actually there; imagery can spread itself across the body like a wave in the ocean, and thus influence all the tissues. The very thought of moving the arm changes the muscle tone of the corresponding muscles. Repetition creates change. If, for example, the image of a soft neck is applied again and again, with time softness will emerge in the tissues of the neck. The more exciting and varied our imagery, and the more the senses are employed, the greater the effect on the body.

Soft neck imagery

1. The neck muscles melting like a sugar cube in warm tea.

2. The neck muscles flowing like a clear mountain brook.

3. The tension in the neck crumbling like a soft cookie on your tongue.

4. The neck muscles melting like vanilla ice cream in the sun.

5. Your own image.

The kinesthetic key

The previous description makes everything sound easy. This is not always the case. Once we have decided that we want to change our bodies, to become more flexible and limber, or improve posture and muscle tone, our old habits may resist with great stubbornness. They are familiar, and we have managed to get through life so far this way. Many are quick to say, "I can't feel anything!" when they first work with imagery, and thus think they are doing something wrong. This is not true: the power of imagery has to be practiced first. It is only with intense use that images start to gain a foothold in the body.

The kinesthetic key, as I call it, is crucial to transforming naked words into images and experiences. Many people have a naturally well-developed sense, while others have to build it up by diligently stoking new feelings like the first sparks of a fire. Later, when images have become part of our extended repertoire, we will be able to activate them. This key is greatly supported in its development by a strong mental presence during practice sessions. This provides our nervous system with a better chance of taking on new patterns. This is why our motto is not "practice makes perfect," but "conscious practice creates new movement behavior." My advice to beginners in imagery is: "don't worry if it doesn't work at first." Like children, we can progress from pretending the imagery is true, to actually experiencing it in our body, and this path will be slightly different for everybody.

Building up resources

The kinesthetic key is based on the resources of our imagery. Our memory, our touch, and keen powers of observation will be crucial to developing the key. Here too, the child-like approach will help. We can rediscover the fascination for all things living and moving: the pacing of the panther in the zoo, weighted, regular and smooth, can hold our attention as if we were seven years old. Leaves glittering in the evening light, swaying and flickering like fire; a school of fish, scattering in star-shaped patterns like underwater fireworks—all will be stored by our brain cells as inspiring raw material for our imagery.

Stroke the belly of a cat and imagine that your back muscles are as soft. Feel the wind on your skin and imagine that this breeze is blowing softly through your bones and organs. While swimming, feel the water gliding over your body. Later, out of the water, remember this feeling and imagine water gliding gently down your skin.

Most people have stored many kinesthetic experiences from their childhood that can serve as important resources. These kinds of experiences are very formative, and the more intense and pleasant such a kinesthetic experience, the more effective the corresponding image will be. A warm refreshing bath might be one original kinesthetic experience.

Drawings, photos, and an experience in nature can serve as kinesthetic inspiration:.

1. Imagine that your shoulders are as light as clouds.

2. Imagine that your head sits upon the spine as softly as a buoy on water as in the picture.

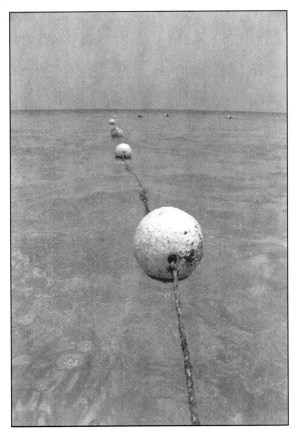

3. Imagine that you are able to float like the woman in the picture.

4. Touch imaginary leaves with your toes.

5. Imagine gliding through water like a seal.

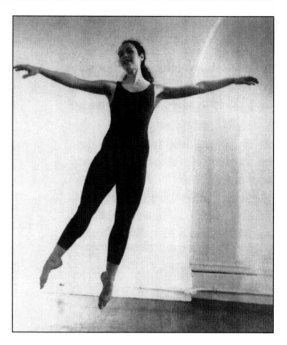

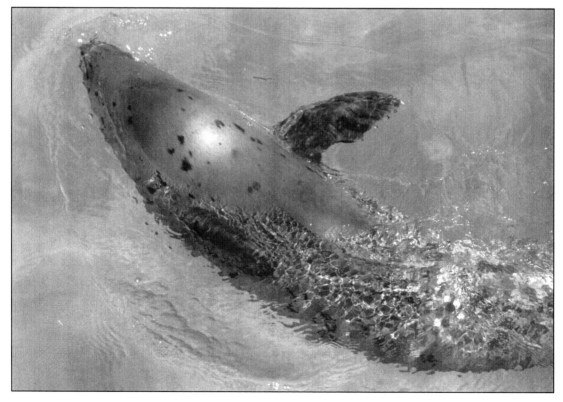

Imagining with all the senses

I believe that our tremendous potential for self-healing is hardly used. One hope I have for this book is that it will show that human beings can be enormously adaptable and self-healing, if only we start to develop the mental muscle of imaging. It is important that we use all our senses as much as possible. Here are of some of the possibilities:

1. Seeing: images can be directly related to the body (my head floats upward), or be a simile (my head floats upward like a balloon).

2. Feeling: either supported by touching (I feel someone massage my shoulders with his hands) or purely kinesthetic (I feel a pleasant breath of wind under my shoulder blades).

3. Hearing: I hear the sound of being in a shower with warm water pouring over my neck, shoulders and back, releasing all the tension.

4. Tasting: I'm standing on a cliff and taste the salty air from the ocean on my tongue.

5. Smelling: I am gently surrounded by the soft scent of roses.

Walking in the forest

In this exercise you will want to make use of all your senses during the visualization: imagine that you are walking through a forest. You can feel the leafy ground underneath your feet, hear the songs of birds and rustling of trees; a ray of light touches your face, and the scent of resin fills your nostrils. You touch a tree. You can feel the roughness of the bark and a slightly sticky spot under a fingertip; a thousand tiny pieces of information are stored in your sensory memory. You touch a leaf and feel its surface as precisely as possible. How do the veins run? Can you feel tiny hairs or a pointy tip?

Try to list all the colors that you can see in the forest. How many sounds do you hear? How does your foot land on the forest floor? How does the atmosphere feel on your cheek? Picture a tree root, and visualize balancing on it. Can you run through the forest? Jump across a brook? See an animal? Stop, breathe and touch a clump of moss. How deeply do your fingers sink into the mossy surface?

The adaptable brain

At birth, our movement skills are very primitive compared to what we are able to do as adults. The ability to carry out complex movement sequences is learned as we grow up. In childhood, we discover, with great joy and unflagging energy, increasingly challenging movements. The words of my six year-old daughters, as we were trying out jumping games and somersaults, still resound in my ears: "Show me something! Show me something new! Show me something else!" Certain reflexes and original movement-patterns influence the development of coordination, but to a large extent our movement learning is controlled by our ability to imitate.

I sometimes used to do pirouettes in our living room (it helped my posture), and my daughter, seeing me, would do threefold pirouettes without having been directly taught. If children didn't have the example of their parents walking on two feet, they would probably not learn to walk. A very different picture can be found with non-human animals. They are born quite finished, as far as movement is concerned. Many mammals can walk on their day of birth. But we are ahead of animals in another way: our diversity. A dolphin knows only how to swim; a horse knows only how to walk on four legs (except in the circus); monkeys prefer to work their way along with their hands, even though they have the ability to walk on their hind legs (albeit with the support of their hands). A human child, on the other hand, shows a great diversity of movement early on: swimming, crawling on all fours, walking on two legs, climbing a tree and modeling a piece of clay with his fingers. This diversity of movement challenges the brain; it has to have variants of control at its disposal, and it has to be able to change quickly from swimming to climbing and back to clay modeling. In other words, our brain has to be adaptable. It is not like a computer, but rather like a plant which needs care, and which thrives better when it is in harmony with its surroundings.

I therefore believe that a lack of *diversity* of movement, and therefore a lack of challenge for the brain, is one of the most important reasons for the problems people increasingly have with their locomotor system. Those who do not challenge themselves are deprived of a vital opportunity for healing and prevention of pain. Consequently, many of the brain's abilities are extinguished, like a fire without fuel.

The most tragic case is probably the back. No part of the body has as many joints as the spine, and so a certain amount of imaginative diversity in movement is called for. And that is just what may be missing in most training programs for the back: a carefully planned and safe, yet diverse set of exercises which train the back and the mind to become more adaptable.

Movement coordination and childhood

A large repertoire of well-coordinated and regularly practiced movements enables you to maintain a movement-oriented, flexible body and mind. Those who move in a wooden, rigid way are not doing anything wrong; they are just missing out on other ways to coordinate movement, and this will eventually cause problems. Being able to span the range of movements from rigid to very flexible is healthy for everyone, not just for the dancer who is trained to exhibit great movement variety. In many cultures, this variety is constantly enriched. I remember a scene from a film about a village in Africa: when someone came to visit the village, all the inhabitants—young and old, men and women—came running, jumping up and down, wriggling with joy. Such behavior would be seen as strange by Western societies! We don't greet people in public by jumping up and down and shaking our bodies, even though it would be a great way to shed weight! (Even though weight loss is a popular goal, I do not think that jumping up and down to greet people will catch on any time soon.) In parts of Africa, dance accompanies people throughout their lives; each phase of life is celebrated with dancing.

For one Cuban folk dancer I know, dance is air, earth and water. But when someone asks him about his profession, upon answering "I dance," he has then been asked: "and what do you do during the day?" The movement arts are, for many adults, an exotic extra, and at best thought of as leisure activities or an activity for young children at the local ballet school. As children we were all artists: we painted, sang, played theater, danced, and drew. Child–rearing without the arts is unthinkable. Yet for many adults these things lose importance; they don't belong to an "honest" or adult way of earning one's living, until perhaps the day they pop up again in creative management seminars or personal development courses.

Childhood movements

Sit down comfortably and try to remember your childhood. Can you remember how you used to move? Can you remember what you especially liked to do? Which games, which movements, made you happy? Do you remember a movement that you would like to try? Romp around in your imagery as you used to. Climb a tree, wade through mud, throw a ball at a wall, drive your bike over a bumpy road, jump through a meadow with high grass, swim in a cool lake, dance a ring-around-the-roses, play catch! Are there movements from your childhood that you would like to bring back into your present life? Be brave, try them out now, and you will feel wonderful thereafter!

Widening our range

In the following section we will find out how to widen our movement repertoire. On one hand, we will discover new movements, and on the other learn how to rid ourselves of harmful movement habits. Movement habits are also called movement patterns. If these patterns are one-dimensional, they can result in damage to the locomotor system. For example, if we use our legs in an unbalanced way, we can shift our pelvis, leading to back problems.

The varying strength of the two legs

Imagine you are in front of a chair, just before sitting down. Move the right leg backward, then sit down and stand up again. Do it once more, but slowly and leisurely, without letting yourself fall onto the seat. This is not as easy, but it is healthier for the back. Stand up and prepare to sit down again by moving the left leg backwards. Again, move slowly, and without letting yourself fall at the end. Did you notice a difference sitting down with the right or left leg? Maybe you noticed that sitting down was easier with one of the legs. This is the leg that is better trained, as it is used to braking your fall when you sit down. This braking action of the thighs and gluteal (buttock) muscles is called *eccentric action*, and it builds up a great deal of strength. If the muscles of one leg are significantly stronger than the muscles of the other, the pelvis may become distorted.

The training effect of daily life

We all sit down many times a day, perhaps a few hundred times per month. This sitting action has a substantial training effect as it carries almost the whole weight of the upper body, from about ninety to one hundred thirty pounds, up and down. This could be good exercise, except that the movement is so one-dimensional, using primarily one leg. This difference in strength between the legs causes unequal muscle development on the two sides of the pelvis. The consequence is that the pelvis becomes slanted and distorted. As the pelvis is the foundation of the spine, it too will be affected. Often the spine tries to compensate for pelvic imbalance, and that will in time cause pain. One then treats the spine as if it were the cause, instead of recognizing the problem in our one-sided movement patterns.

As in the example above, our movement habits exercise certain muscles more than others. One of our legs has a considerable lead in strength, and on top of that becomes further developed with daily use.

The solution? We could simply strengthen the weak leg more, but to find the right balance we must train both legs together. Even if we try to balance them with work-out and with stretching techniques, one-sided patterns will be reinforced in daily life.

As long as we don't change the patterns, our training will be one-sided. The best solution is to discover and then re-balance your movement patterns in daily life. The key is the intelligent observation of your own body. You observe your body in order to learn where you can improve, just like a gardener watching his plants grow decides which have been watered too much or too little. It makes more sense to achieve balance with your "movement feeling" than to try to correct each muscle. If you stretch or tone a muscle with the goal of correcting an imbalance, without changing the awareness of the joint, then you will quickly fall back into old patterns. But if you start to move in a balanced fashion, the muscles will adapt to this.

As soon as you have attained a new "movement feeling," it is crucial that you are aware when the old habits are trying to creep in again. When do I pull my shoulders up again? In what situations do I tense my back? Hold my breath? Like a watchdog, you have to scrutinize and catch yourself immediately. Only then have you truly conquered the old pattern and given the new pattern priority over the old.

Sometimes we make the embarrassing discovery that we are very attached to old patterns even though they are obviously not healthy. We don't want to give them up, even if they cause pain. The image we have of our body is interwoven with the old pattern to such a degree that we have a hard time accepting the world without pain and tension. It feels as if something old and dear were missing. In my classes, I have often seen others experience this. Obviously the participants arrive in class with the desire for relaxed shoulders and a tension-free back; but if this state is achieved, one does not see only happy faces—much to my astonishment. A puzzled look shows that this is all rather strange, and in conversation during the next break, the shoulders are pulled back up toward the ears.

For the change to become permanent, the new experience must be integrated into the present body image. If tension has been our way of life for ten years, then relaxation and effortless movement seem odd, even if our intellect tells us they are not good for us. In order to accept a new movement pattern as our own, we need to repeat the process that got us there over and over again, until the new feeling is normal and the old one uncomfortable. Relaxation, or any change in the body, consists of psychological as well as physical adjustments. As long as our feelings of identity and security are based on a certain amount of tension, we will not be able to move loosely and unencumbered in daily life.

One of my workshop participants came to me with chronic hand tension that he wanted to relieve. After a few exercises with imagery and movement his hands had become limber and flexible, and he said, "Oh! My hands are totally relaxed—but these are not my hands!"

Self-observation in daily life

1. Observe yourself in daily life: How do I move? How do I breathe? What do I do in a one-sided way? Do I hold my head forward, to the back, always to one side? When do I overly tense my muscles?

2. When I take a step, which leg leads?

3. Which leg do I step on first when I go up the stairs? Observe yourself going up and down stairs.

4. How do I dry myself after showering? How do I hold the towel?

5. To which side do I turn when I spontaneously look behind me or turn around in bed?

6. Do I tense or pull up one shoulder when I get up or sit down?

Building up new movement patterns

1. From this book, choose exercises that appeal to you and practice them every day.

2. Discover new possibilities in the body. To achieve this you can use imagery, movement, the touch of a partner, and the pictures in this book. Some of the pictures can help you recognize your patterns, and others serve as inspiration for building new ones.

3. Give new habits a chance by imagining and thinking about them as often as possible. The brain is like a recording machine. It records what you think, imagine, and how you move, and tends to replay them.

4. Practice balanced, tension-free movement, and this is what the brain will start recording and playing. The nervous system needs to have the opportunity to establish the new possibilities. At first it may only be "as if;" later it will become real experience.

5. Notice when you fall back into the old patterns.

6. Accept newly gained relaxation and movement patterns in daily life as normal.

7. Try to approach the whole thing as a game in which you can always laugh at yourself. Don't be discouraged if it doesn't work right away!

Constructive Rest

We have seen that it isn't easy to change noxious movement patterns. As soon as we move again, we are using precisely those patterns that we want to change, therefore reinforcing them even more. Compare the situation to two competing speaker systems: in order to hear sound from the first system, the second one has to be turned down. Transferring this image into movement means that new, more efficient movement patterns have to step into the foreground, while the old ones fade into the background. That is why Mabel Todd, founder of ideokinetic imagery systems, suggested exercising with images in a lying-down position, which she named the *Constructive Rest Position* (CRP). Because we aren't moving, old movement patterns can't be activated. Even sitting or standing can activate those old patterns and distract our movement control with old information. The new patterns

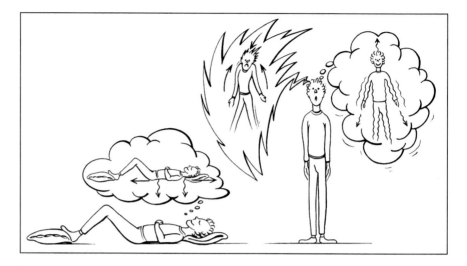

cannot easily assert themselves under these circumstances (as in accompanying illustration).

Here is an example: let's say you tend to have a hollow back while standing. So you try to visualize the back muscles relaxing and the pelvis straightening itself, but the old patterns dominate too strongly and not much changes. Then you exercise in the Constructive Rest Position, and visualize the back muscles relaxing. There will be almost no interference from the old patterns, and the new patterns have a chance of becoming integrated. Furthermore, you have gravity and the ground as allies. Gravity pulls your hollow back downward, and the ground pushes the pelvis up: both help to improve your posture.

I find it very helpful, right after practicing in the lying position, to integrate new images into the movements of daily life; I use new insight achieved in the CRP to help me experience these new patterns, and to integrate them into my body image.

Lying down comfortably

The most important rule of the Constructive Rest Position, or Constructive Rest, is lying in a comfortable position. If you are not lying down comfortably, you're not able to concentrate on the images. Suggestions for a comfortable position are as follows:

1. Many people lie better if the knees are bent at about ninety degrees with the soles of the feet on the ground. This is because of shortened hip joint flexors which connect the thigh bone with the pelvis. When the legs are stretched straight, a hollow back posture can occur (it is possible to have Constructive Rest with stretched legs.) As Constructive Rest changes our posture due to gravity, it helps us to stretch the back and minimize the hollow back (see illustration). When we stand up, gravity has the effect of compressing our spine; when we lie down, the spine stretches again.

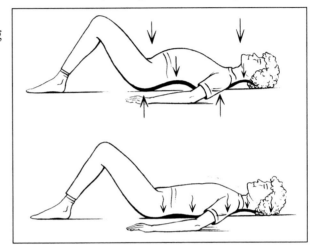

2. To stop your legs from falling sideways, you can bind them together with a soft cloth a little above the knee.

3. A small cushion under the balls of the feet and under the head is more comfortable for most people. A cushion under the head is indispensable if one has a large thorax or generally bends the head forward a lot when standing up.

4. A small cushion under the pelvis or two cushions next to the pelvis are sometimes helpful, too.

5. Constructive Rest can also be practiced very well with a partner supporting your imagery with touch (see illustration).

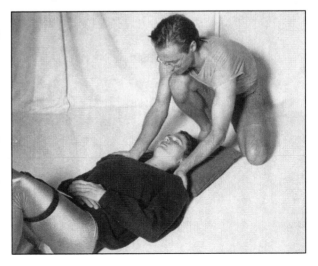

6. After Constructive Rest, put your arms around your knees and rock

the body back and forth a little, imagining that the back is expanding like bread dough. Visualize the hip fold as being very deep and soft.

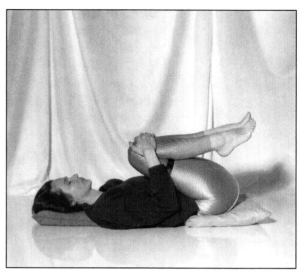

7. Before getting up, roll to your side and gently tap your back with your uppermost hand. If you have a partner, let him or her gently stroke or tap your back before you get up (see illustration).

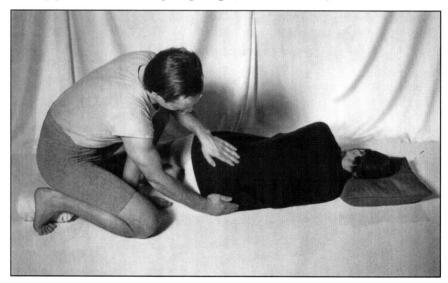

8. Constructive Rest can be accompanied by calming music.

Thoughts on Constructive Rest

1. If you anticipate the result of an exercise, you are depriving yourself of the chance to discover something new. In other words, just visualize the images without having any expectations.

2. Visualized movement is enough. In CRP, we don't do any active movements; otherwise we may just activate old movement patterns.

3. Don't force yourself to use Constructive Rest. If you feel like lying down, this is a good moment for CRP; if you feel like a walk in the woods then that is what you should do.

4. Becoming older can mean experiencing inner movement less and less. However, movement imagery can rejuvenate us. In CRP we experience movement inside the body. All images should therefore be moving images.

5. Creativity means having the courage to start something new, and also to have the courage to change what one has started. In CRP we open up new territories in the body by using imagery and curiosity.

Constructive Rest: water

Visualize lying at the beach on very soft sand. It feels very pleasant to sink softly into the sand. Look at the indentation your body has left in the sand. Mentally trace the edge of this indentation and visualize its outline. Feel the depth of the indentation in the sand. How deeply do the back of the head, shoulders, arms, back, buttocks, and feet lie in the sand? Now imagine that your back is spreading out in the sand. It spreads like a wave rippling over the beach. Feel your back: warm, soft and flowing (see illustration). Feel the movement of

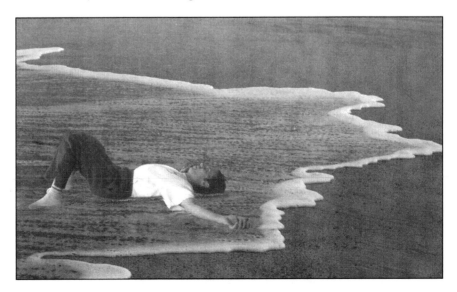

your back as it expands. The water takes all your tension away as it flows back into the sea. It flows along your back, between the *spinous processes* and the ribs, loosening all the tension. Water flushes through the insides of your body. The structure of your bones looks like a honeycomb with many cavities. Feel these spaces being cleansed and loosened.

Spacious and light,

Open spaces in our bones,

Water cleansing our bones.

A breath of wind on the sea

Brings air and light

Into the depths of our body.

Our eyes are liquid containers:

The eyes

Are filled with crystal-clear water,

Carried in soft hollows.

The hollow of the eye is spacious,

There is space for creative sight.

To loosen the shoulders we liberate

The shoulder blade from the thorax:

A soft cushion is placed between the shoulder blade and the thorax.

The cushion fluffs up, fills out the space.

The shoulder blade rests on the pillow

Away from the thorax.

Constructive Rest: dialogue with the body

There are things our body knows that haven't yet reached our consciousness. By asking the body questions with great openness, and without any expectations, we can find out much about our inner state.

1. Observe your breathing for a few minutes.

2. Let your inner eye roam around the body for a bit. Take your time; the inner eye is in no hurry.

3. Look at the thorax, pelvis, head, arms, hands, legs and feet from the inside.

4. Then ask yourself if there is a place your inner eye is attracted to. Is there a spot that you want to look at more closely? There will be no obvious logic behind the spot chosen by the inner eye.

5. Ask this spot: "Is there something I can do for you? Is there something I should know or feel?" Wait calmly for an answer.

6. The answer may not fit your expectations. It could manifest itself as a word, an image, feeling, a sound, or an urge to do a certain movement.

7. If you notice that your mind has strayed from your body, observe your breathing once more. Then observe which spot in your body your inner eye is drawn to and again ask the question: "What can I do for you?" Wait for an answer.

8. When the answering process is finished, you can observe where the inner eye is now, or note your experiences and images in your diary.

Constructive Rest: heaviness and lightness

The experience of weight and heaviness is crucial for relaxation. Often it is enough to feel weight in a certain part of the body in order to free it of tension. The counterpart to weight is the feeling of lightness. Lightness is experienced in relation to weight. In a tense muscle, both the feeling of weight and lightness are missing. In the next exercise using Constructive Rest we will concentrate on both weight and lightness.

1. Lie down in the CRP and observe your breathing.

2. Realize that you can decide at any moment which thoughts you want to have flicker across your inner screen, and which ones not to.

3. Decide to take full control over your inner screen. If any distracting thoughts come up, imagine them melting and dissolving. Say

to yourself that each thought is destined to melt—and soon you will have a calm mind.

4. Visualize the cells of your body. Each cell has a top and a bottom.

5. Each cell has its lower part turned toward the earth; feel its heaviness, its weight. Each cell also has an upper part, turned toward heaven. This has a feeling of lightness.

6. Allow each of your cells to be carried by gravity. Don't try to keep them up off the surface of the earth; let them sink downward.

7. Your cells are also flexible in relation to each other; they can glide in their heaviness around one another. They have a flexible heaviness.

8. Feel the heaviness of the cells in your neck. Feel how they sink, allowing themselves to be pulled toward the earth. Feel how they glide around one another.

9. Feel the weight in the cells of your shoulders. Feel how they sink toward the earth, and how they glide around each other.

10. Feel the weight of the cells in your lumbar spine. Feel how they sink, falling toward the earth, and how they glide around one another.

11. Feel the weight of the cells wherever you are tense at the moment.

12. Feel that your cells also have a certain kind of lightness so that they can move from heaviness to lightness.

13. Stand up and feel the weight, the heaviness and lightness of your cells.

Constructive Rest: the bones and muscles

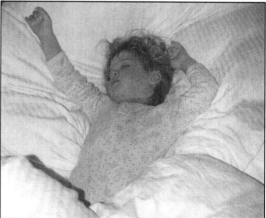

In many people, the muscles surrounding the bones are like a bodice that is too-tightly laced. This has serious consequences for quality of movement, and restricts the joints in their natural freedom of movement. In the next CRP exercise and the following movement improvisation, we will try to free up these two important structures of the body:

1. Lie down in the CRP and observe your breathing. Visualize your bones resting in the in the cushiony, downy bed of your muscles. What does it mean to rest, to really give yourself up to resting? Your bones rest like the completely relaxed sleep of a child.

2. Visualize the muscles enveloping the bones. Like a silk summer dress, the muscles fall over the bones. A gentle breeze is enough to make the muscles swing loosely around the bones.

3. Move with these two thoughts: (1) the bones move the muscles; (2) the muscles move the bones. Which image do you prefer?

Constructive Rest: relaxation of the nerves

1. Put two Franklin balls* (see Appendix, page 130) under your buttocks and make soft rocking movements with the pelvis.

2. Put your hands on your belly and feel your organs falling onto your back, like leaves falling from a tree to the ground.

3. Feel the rocking movement calming your organs like a mother calming her baby.

4. Allow both your superficial and your deep belly muscles to relax. The belly rises and sinks slowly with the movement of your breathing.

5. Imagine the many nerves in this area floating as if suspended in water. (See illustration on the following page). With your mind's eye, gaze calmly at these nerves. Your gaze tells the nerves that it is time to rest, that it is time to just "be."

6. Feel the nerves sinking down, resting on the bottom of the belly next to the spine, deep inside the body.

7. Think to yourself: "There is nothing that needs to be done; there is only rest."

8. Take the balls away and notice the sensations in your back. Your back may feel more relaxed and spread on the floor.

9. Take plenty of time to get up from the floor.

---

* Franklin balls are about six inches in diameter and made of springy plastic. They can be ordered from Orthopedic Physical Therapy Products (www.optp.com) in the US.

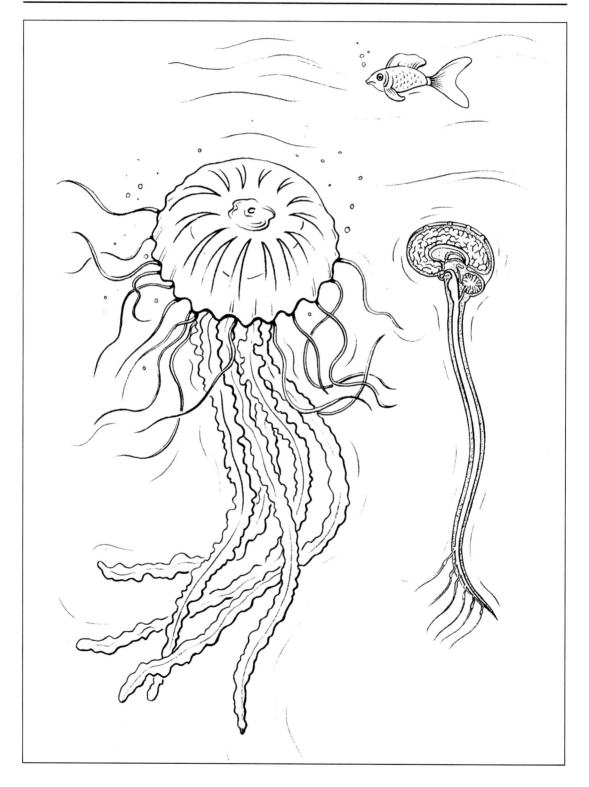

4 The Posture

Good posture is flexible and free and moves without effort. If one has a good posture, one doesn't think about it; it just is. If posture training is based on forcing oneself into a certain position then this artificial posture will remain only as long as effort is used to keep it up. Posture training is only of any use if it helps us to move economically and loosely. A posture which doesn't allow itself to be translated into quality of movement is merely a superficial holding pattern. Dynamic posture and quality of movement are two sides of the same coin.

As soon as you have tightened up in any way for the sake of an improved posture—lifting the thorax and pulling in the belly—you have made movement more difficult. Moving requires contraction of the muscles. If the muscles are already contracted to maintain a certain posture, you will not be able to move very well.

A relaxed and tension-free posture should not be confused with weakness. In blockbuster movies, the hero hurls his opponent through the air with relatively stiff arms and little movement in the spine: the popular image of strength is of high tension. But behind the scenes, the masseur is already waiting to avert the impending lumbago; even the most muscle-loaded body can't be strong without being flexible. On the other hand the comparatively delicate figure of the oriental martial arts practitioner tends to surprise when he or she can easily split a stack of bricks with one blow. Looseness isn't weakness, rather, it is being prepared to move in any given way.

The primary and the secondary skeletons

The skeleton can be divided into a pre-evolution older part and its subsequent evolutionary modification, the younger part. The older part contains the spine, the ribs and the skull, excluding the jaw. This corresponds to the structure of the early vertebrates, in which the spine and thorax dominated and there was no jaw. Millennia later, arms, and with them the shoulder blades as well as the legs and two pelvic wings, became more fully developed. Knowing this can help improve our posture and flexibility, since we tend to weaken the primary skeleton and create tension in the secondary one. In other words, the extremities try to compensate for the lack of strength in the axis and center of the human body.

In an adult, spinal movement usually follows the movement of the arms and legs. But this was not always the case: infants use their spines in an intense and varied fashion before the limbs are very active or controlled. Before they are able to use their arms and legs for support, they are able to crawl on their stomachs like a caterpillar. This rather slow mode of locomotion is very important in developing strength, as every vertebral joint is exercised, massaged, and lubricated. Most adults have a reduced ability to move their individual vertebrae because many of us do not practice varied movements of our spines daily. The whole is only as strong as the sum of its parts, so how can one expect the spine to be strong if the movement of its parts is limited? Workouts for the stomach and back muscles must be accompanied by spinal agility, so as to not increase pressure on the vertebral disks and joints.

Snaky spine movement

1. Put two Franklin balls under the pelvis and two under the upper back. (Tennis balls are not suitable as they are too small and too hard.)

2. Place a pillow under the head.

3. Let your body sink onto the balls. Now start to make slow snake-like movements with the spine.

4. Try to use every part of the spine.

5. After about five minutes, take the balls away and see what feels different about your spine. Can you transfer this feeling to sitting, standing and walking?

Improvisation: spine veil dance

Imagine your body as a loose veil that surrounds the spine (see illustration on the following page). Choose some music that inspires you to move, and imagine that all your movements originate from the spine. Your arms swing with the music because your spine swings;

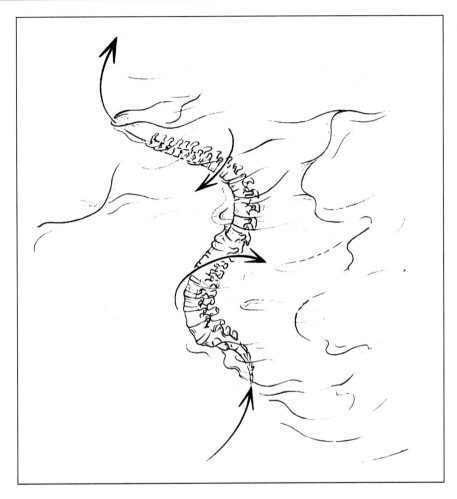

your legs swing because your spine has initiated it; your thorax twists because the spine twisted first. The whole body is a loose silken cloth that follows the swinging movements of the spine.

Your brain and nervous system are in constant dialogue with every part of your body; you could not move otherwise. So why not speak to your spine? Ask your spine what movement it recommends to improve its health. Say: "dear spine, what can I do for you today? Is there any movement you would like to do?" The answer might come as an impulse to move in a fashion you have never moved before, or to do an exercise for your back. The spine knows something about being a spine. It knows what movement it needs; if you trust it, you will discover this movement. Just by reading these words you will notice a certain urge to move your spine; it becomes rather difficult to just sit and read quietly, and your spine will begin to stir and at least adjust itself slightly. This is the spine's own movement voice slowly waking up.

How are you?

Considering the immense variety of bodily feelings we can experience from extreme pain to great pleasure, the answers we provide when someone asks us how we are, are mostly rather neutral. "How are you?" is usually answered by "fine," "OK," "great," "coming along." You will not hear: "my breath is deep and relaxed today, and my spine feels long and flexible!," or "today all my joints really feel elastic and well lubricated," or "my shoulders and neck are so relaxed today, it's wonderful." Such statements are rarely heard; if someone elaborates on his or her health, it will most likely be in the negative: "my back is killing me today!," or "my feet hurt."

Now these things may or may not be true, but by voicing only the negative, we strengthen the negative. To experience the power of expressing yourself in a positive manner about your body, try the following exercise: for one day, always say something positive about your body when someone greets you. If you are too shy to do this, just think your positive answer and don't worry about being overly positive to start with. If you truly do this all day long, you will feel the difference in your body.

Why the spine is curved

In contrast to that of animals, the human spine is not horizontally but vertically aligned. High up at the end of a long curved column sits a rather heavy head (approximately eleven pounds). This offers many advantages: we can keep an overview of our surroundings, we can change directions quickly, and we can see further into the distance than our former rivals from the animal kingdom. Advance planning, not brute force, was crucial to humans thousands of years ago, and still is.

Because of its central position, the spine is key to our posture. In order for it to function well, it needs a healthy, balanced double-S curve. Viewed from the side, we can see two places that are concave, and two places that are slightly arched or convex. The two concave areas are the *cervical* and *lumbar lordosis* of the spine, and the two convex ones are the *thoracic* and *sacrum-coccygeal kyphosis* of the spine. The whole forms a double-S shape which, when in a balanced state, holds many advantages for effortless movement, If, however, the head is not balanced properly, but held forward, for example, the spinal column is unbalanced and muscular effort is increased. For a short period of time this is not a problem, but after weeks, months, or years of overwork, the muscles and joints are screaming for relief.

Why is the spine a double S? (See illustrations **a** – **d**.) Would it not be easier if we had a straight column (**a**)? Actually, a straight central column would be advantageous if we didn't have to move, since with movement it would quickly become strained (**b**). Furthermore, with a straight spine, it would be difficult to find space for the thorax containing the lungs and heart. Thanks to the curves in our spine, the center of the thorax can be situated above our support area, reducing muscular effort. For women giving birth, a straight spine would provide only a very limited space in the pelvis for the baby and its descent through the birth canal. The steeply forward-tilted sacrum in women affords a more spacious exit for the baby. A single-S would distribute our weight too far from the center of the body, and would hinder the flow of forces through the spine (**c**). Furthermore, several curves in combination are stronger than a single one (**d**). For the proper functioning of a column of curves, the areas where weight is moved from one direction to the other are crucial. Just as a car is more likely to go off the road on a curve, those places in the spine experience the most gravity. To keep the curves of the spine in balance is thus central to the well-being of the back.

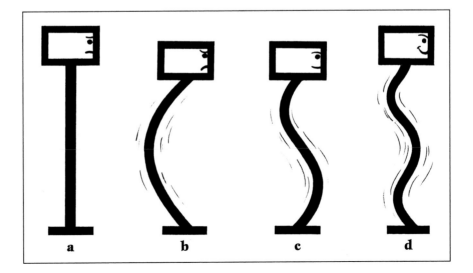

a   b   c   d

How did this all come about? As mankind changed posture from a four-legged, horizontal, spined mammal, the spine was reconfigured and now has a completely different relationship with gravity. For the human body to be balanced, individual weights need to be balanced over each other. As we can observe in the spine of our closest relative, the chimpanzee, whose spine is further back in the body, early man had to bring his spine closer to the center. Several things happened during evolution. The top of the sacrum, which forms the base of the lumbar spine, was bent forward to bring it underneath the mass of weight hovering above it. The spine was also rather deep-set, and the ribs became angled backward significantly before curving

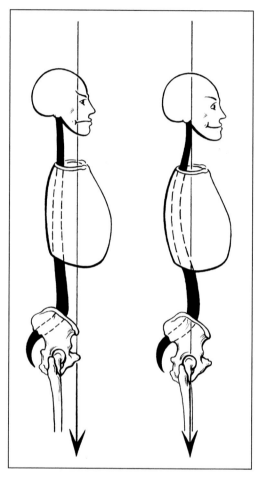

forward to close the thorax in front. The double-S curve also served to bring much of the mass of the spine further forward. The spine now occupies a much more central position in the body.

The spine as a wave

The spine originated out of ocean creatures' desire to be able to move with purpose and not just by pure chance. The spine created a front and a back for the animal, a direction from where it came, and to where it could go. Animals with spines originated in the water, though at this point they may have moved with wavy motions, and their spines did not have a fixed wave shape built into them as ours does. A fast animal, especially in the cat family, may make wave-like movements in its spine to lengthen its running stride, but in no animals are waves fixed into the basic shape of the spine. Not even humans are born with a wave shaped spine; this shape is developed through movement and practice, through the child's efforts to crawl, sit, walk, and run.

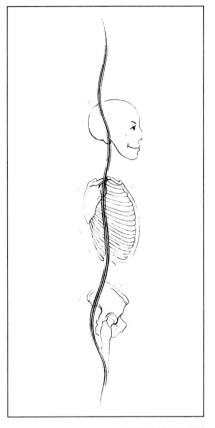

I like to think that perhaps after millions of years of living among the waves, our cells have formed a spine modeled after the image of the wave. The human spine looks like a snapshot of a wave. It would be of great advantage if everyone could bring the sense of flow to the spine. In fact, each step we take creates a small wave that rises from the bottom to the top of our spine (see illustration at right). Unfortunately, many spines look and feel as if the wave was frozen solid. Our task is to keep the spinal waves fluid and mobile throughout our lives.

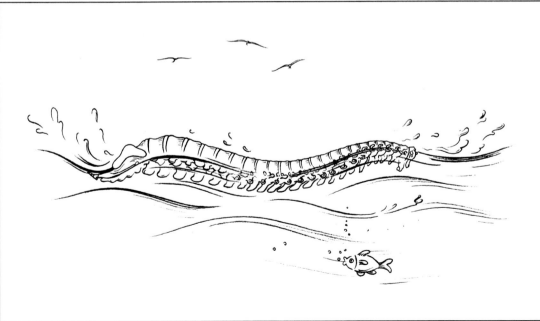

Vertebral body and disk

The inner part of the spine, pointing towards the belly, consists of the round vertebral bodies and disks. The outer part of the spine consists of the vertebral *foramen* of the spinal cord and spinous processes, which radiate backward and sideways. These processes are points of attachment for muscles and ligaments, presenting a complex structure of struts and elastic elements of traction. This enables the spine to be very flexible and to keep its shape at the same time. The spine has many joints with small flat facets that in the lumbar spine permit easy flexion and extension, while in the thoracic spine they are arranged to allow for bending to the side and rotation.

The bodies of the vertebrae and the disks are designed to carry weight, while the joints of the spine are designed to be free to create movement. Astonishingly, healthy disks can handle more weight than the bony vertebral bodies (the disks and vertebral bodies transfer ninety percent of the upper body's weight through the spine). Nevertheless, these basically sturdy disks sometimes have a negative image. This is not surprising: what do you think about a place for which only bad news is heralded? Complaints of slipped disks are commonplace, but rarely does anyone speak about their strong and healthy disks, disks that are in the right place at the right time.

To make things worse, it seems the fashionable way to stand and gesture is in a rather slumped and bent-over way, compressing the spine. What is trendy posture for young adults is a disaster for the disks. Look at mannequins in window displays for more examples of disk-compressing postures.

Some claim that the spine, and especially the disks, are the weak spots of the human motor system, having evolved too rapidly from the horizontal to the vertical position. Considering that upright gait has been around for at least nine million years, there seems to have been ample time for evolution. It is better to think that weakness lies in our posture and movement behavior rather than in our physical make-up. If one moves regularly and economically in a variety of ways, and the disks are relieved from time to time, they will remain healthy. Problems surface when the disks are not nourished properly due to tension in the muscles and organs.

Strength training may improve the force of the spinal muscles, but doesn't necessarily change movement habits. Certainly the spine will be more stabilized after months and years of strength training but its postural weaknesses will be reinforced. Think of the lean-

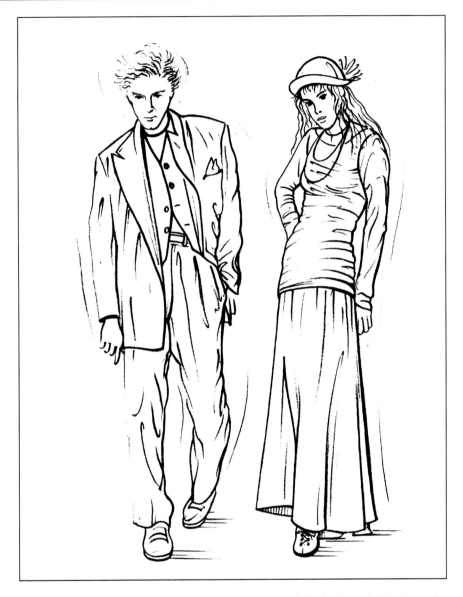

ing tower of Pisa. It is still leaning. Even while it is stabilized with more and more supports (like muscles), it is only a question of time until the tower collapses.

Our goal is to create a healthy spine through movement and a relaxed posture. We do not want to look for a stop-gap solution, but to find out which habits lie at the root of our back problems, and change them.

Our workouts will become more effective if we not only train our muscles but also foster healthy movement habits. It is not necessary to press the spine against a wall in order to achieve a better posture. Why? Because a wall is not a good role model for the spine. It is rigid, has no curves, cannot usually flex or extend, creating a disadvantageous body feeling and an imagery of stiffness.

To sum up: before and during workouts, become aware of your posture and movement habits, and make sure that they are the best you can manage for the moment. The illustration below demonstrates the following: joints are locked by a tense musculature (**a**); alignment is improved through imagery (**b**); and muscle strength is integrated into a well-coordinated body (**c**) and (**d**).

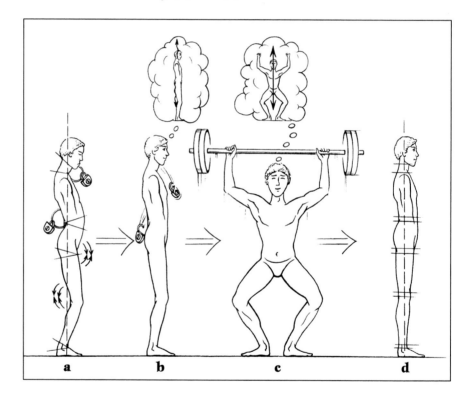

a   b   c   d

Spine and champagne

In the CRP (see page 33), imagine a river flowing up the front side of your spine. When the water has reached the upper end of the thoracic spine, it tumbles like a waterfall down the back of your spine, to the tailbone (*coccyx*), flushing all the tension out of your back. Ask a friend to help you with the above image. With one hand, gently stroke from the front of the pubic bone (*pelvis*) up toward the breastbone to support the feeling of an upward flow. With both hands, stroke downward on the left and right of the back to help the feeling of downward flow.

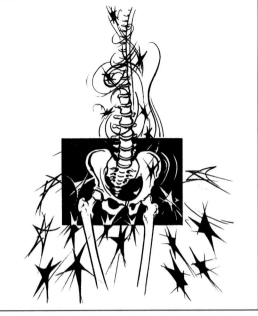

And now an image for partygoers: after imagining the flow of water up and down the spine, roll to one side and tap yourself on your back (in case you don't have a partner) and take some time to stand up. While standing, imagine that champagne (or mineral water) bubbles are rising up the spine. Feel the bubbles caressing the spine, lifting it upwards. The bubbles lead to a feeling of tingling freshness and lift, as if twinkling stars were carrying our spine.

The jaw and spine

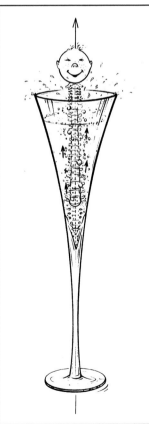

Probably no joint in the body is used more than the joints of the jaw. Just imagine how much we speak and chew during an average day. Whether speaking, eating, or swallowing, the joints of the jaw are in continuous use, not to mention jaw clenching and grinding during a tense moment (to be avoided, of course). How often do we perform actual jaw exercises at the gym (besides chatting with friends)? Usually the jaw is in need of relaxation; tension in the jaw radiates to the spine, affecting breathing and digestion, and can be responsible for headaches, migraines and neck pains. The jaw moves with the help of a complex joint and a disk made of cartilage that lies between the joint socket in the skull (*temporal bone*) and the rounded *condyle* of the jawbone. The disk is a soft but very strong oblong cushion that increases flexibility and maintains the stability of the joint. There are two joints on each side of the disk: an upper joint between the temporal bone and disk, and a lower joint between the disk and jaw joint condyle.

You can find the jaw joint by putting the fingers in the openings of your ears. Now press your fingers forward and move your jaw. What you feel are the condyles, the joint of the jaw in action. If you place your fingers just in front of the ear openings you will be right on top of the jaw joint. Open and close your mouth and feel the jaw joints in action. When you open the mouth wide you can feel the condyle of the jaw moving down and forward beneath your skin. There is a lot of room for movement in this joint. Imagine the jaw is only flexibly connected to the skull. Bend your head to the right and let the jaw fall sideways to the right. Bend your head to the left and let the jaw fall sideways to the left. If you can do this with ease then you have successfully released some tension in your jaw.

Jaw tension and breathing

1. Feel your breathing.

2. Now tense your jaw muscles by pressing the teeth together.

3. For a few moments observe the effect of the tension in the jaw on your breathing.

4. Relax the jaw muscles by opening the mouth slightly and feeling the weight of the jaw. What effect does this have on your breathing? You'll see that releasing tension in your jaw means relief of tension in your breathing.

The gliding disk

The disk can be found between the condyle of the jaw and the skull. When you open your mouth wide, it glides forward like a soft air mattress from under the temporal bone. The "temporal bone slide" is curved like an upside-down playground slide. The disk glides forward

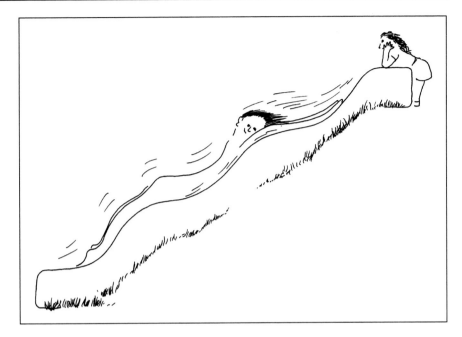

from under the slide (see illustration above). Put your fingers in front of the ear lobes and then move them up a bit: there is the disk. Remember the feeling of going down a slide in the playground? Often the disk doesn't glide equally on both sides: on one side it feels looser. Move your jaw back and forth a bit— maybe it's easier to move the jaw to one side than the other. Move it back and forth again and imagine that the two disks are equally thick and able to glide.

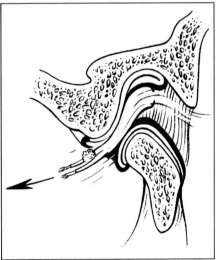

The head turns around the jaw

We tend to visualize the jaw moving from the temporal bone joint. Now we will experience the opposite by imagining that the skull moves, not the jaw. First touch the jaw joint above the ear lobe again; imagine that the skull rests on this joint. Now hold the jaw with both hands and rock the head around the jaw joints. The head is the seesaw and the condyles of the jaw joints are the pivots of this seesaw (see illustration below). The skull swings on the jaw. Anyone who has seen a baby nursing has seen the pumping motion of the skull. The movement of the skull around the jaw causes a small stretching of the neck and back muscles. As adults we tend to keep the head rigid and only move the jaw while eating, no longer feeling the looseness of the skull. The next section will further expand on this topic.

The head sits in the saddle

The position and movement of our head greatly affects our entire posture. If the position of the head is crooked or pushed too far forward or back, then the whole spine is out of balance. Imagine a rider sitting on the head of the horse or hanging from the saddle sideways! If the head is poorly positioned, then the blood vessels and the spinal cord will be compressed where they enter the skull.

The uppermost vertebra is called the *atlas* and has not one but two small saddles next to each other. They look like the hollows of a modern office chair. At the bottom of the skull there are also two protrusions, which we will call the "sitting bones" of the skull. Thus the head sits with its sitting bones on a tailor-made atlas chair.

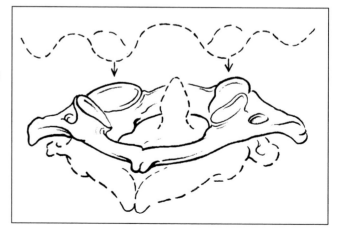

When we sit on a chair, we can feel our weight being transferred onto the seat. We can also concentrate on how the seat carries us: the seat presses up into our buttocks. This is one of Newton's laws of physics: if a force (our weight) pushes against an object (the chair), this will trigger an identical counter force (the chair pushes against our buttocks).

This principle is helpful in optimizing the effects of the various forces in the body. We have just visualized the head sitting in a saddle. Now imagine the facets carrying the head: the facets, the little saddles, push upward with a force that corresponds to the weight of the head. It is important that this force be transferred at this point from the spine onto the head. If this isn't the case, the muscles have to work more, which can lead to tension in the neck. If we manage to imagine the point of weight transfer, then the neck muscles will relax, as the head is now being carried by the joint intended to do that. The muscles are thus free to fulfill their main task: to move the head. A key principle of wellness is: *your flexibility is only as good as your posture.* With poor posture, the muscles are forced to contract, holding on to the imbalanced bones; otherwise the body collapses. As soon as you improve your posture and the way the bones are aligned your muscles are freed and your flexibility improves instantly.

Visualize the muscles at the back of the neck. Weight transfer between the skull and the spine does not take place here; this is the place where movement is generated. Talk to this place with your inner voice: "You can let go, the head is sitting comfortably on the atlas. The head is centered in its saddle." Visualize the nape muscles (at the top of the back of the neck) being light and soft, flowing like water and bubbling like a mountain spring. Also think of the muscles in front of the atlas. Imagine these muscles becoming as soft as a cotton ball. The tongue is one of these muscles. Imagine your tongue as soft as a cloud and permeable, as if it were possible to breathe in and out through the tongue.

The head balances on the atlas

1. Put your fingers behind your ear lobes. There you will find a bony protrusion called the *mastoid process*.

2. Right under the mastoid process are the *transverse processes* of the top vertebra, the atlas. Maybe you can feel these protrusions under the neck muscles.

3. Imagine a line connecting the two mastoid processes. In the

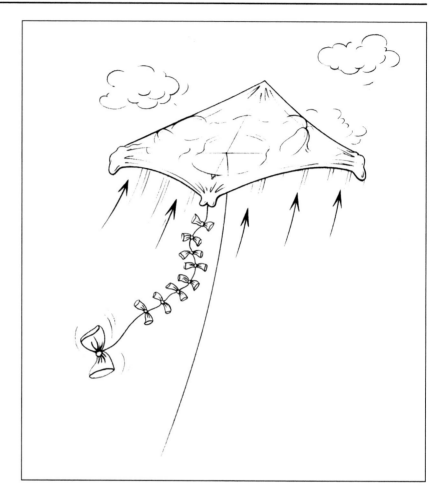

middle of this line are the two sitting bones of the skull and the two hollows of the atlas they fit into.

4. Imagine the head resting evenly on the two hollows. Allow the weight of the head to settle completely into the hollows, which are meant for precisely that. You can support this transfer of weight by exhaling "Ahh," while imagining the head resting on the atlas.

5. Make sure you don't bend the neck while feeling the weight of the head.

6. Rock the head back and forth in the atlas hollows. Try not to bend and stretch the neck, but just to move the head on the joint between it and the top vertebra. Imagine the sitting bones of the head gliding smoothly in the sit hollows of the atlas. Feel the head sitting in the saddle.

Lifting the bone marrow

Considerable pressure can build up in the spinal marrow due to bad posture. In the neck area, and in its spinal marrow, the nervous tissue of the skull is under a lot of pressure through the habitual bending forward of the head. This can cause headaches and dizziness. A very strong protective skin, the *dura mater*, envelops the marrow. It provides some protection, but is easily bent. Within the dura, and around the marrow, the *cerebrospinal fluid* (CSF) is found. The CSF is a liquid that surrounds the brain and spinal cord to nourish and protect it. In a sense, our central nervous system is floating inside the skull and spine. This is a great image, and, with it, we can conjure up a feeling of lightness and ease in all our actions. Try to imagine the dura and the CSF helping us ease our posture.

Imagine the many messages being sent up through the spinal cord to the brain at any moment. These allow you to know where you are in space and to feel your body. Imagine that pleasant movements will, in turn, create pleasant feelings that rise up through your spine. Imagine the dura like a diver's suit for the spinal cord and the brain. Imagine the spinal cord floating within the dura, comfortably protected and buoyed by the warm surrounding fluid.

The iliopsoas muscle

The *iliopsoas* is a muscle located deep within our body between the upper legs and spine. Seventy years ago Mabel Todd discovered the importance of this muscle in posture and movement. The iliopsoas is actually two muscles that attach in the same place. The *psoas* connects the spine and the legs from the lumbar area to the inside top of the thigh. The *iliac* muscle connects the inside of the wings of the pelvis (*ilia*) in the same place on the inside of the upper part of the thigh (see illustration **a** on page 60). If these muscles are weak or tight, they strain the lower back and cause postural problems.

The iliopsoas supporting the spine

Imagine the iliopsoas as supporting hands for the spine, as this is how it feels when the muscle is elongated and strong (see illustration **b** on page 60). The ilipsoas is also our most important hip flexor. We walk, jump, and climb stairs with significant help from this muscle. We will now take a closer look at these two muscles, and discover the central part they play in our posture and for our back.

The origin of the psoas can be found in the disks and the vertebrae of the lumbar region. A muscle that exerts a direct pulling action between disks and legs has to be looked after with special care. Uncoordinated movements of the legs can cause problems for the spine due to a tense, shortened psoas. Unfortunately this muscle is in exactly that state in many people because of hours sitting in a forward slouch. The kidneys rest on the psoas, and the extensive lumbar nerve plexus is located in and around it. After releasing tension in this area, a cozy, relaxed feeling in the lower abdomen develops. There are also connections between the diaphragm and the psoas, so that breathing rhythm is related to walking. This isn't surprising, as breathing and walking evolved at the same time when creatures first came on land.

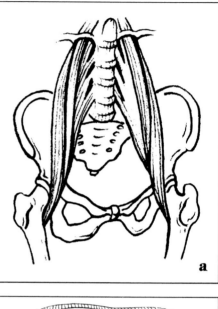

How do tension and contractions of the iliopsoas come about? While we are sitting, the front of the lumbar spine, the origin of the psoas, lies

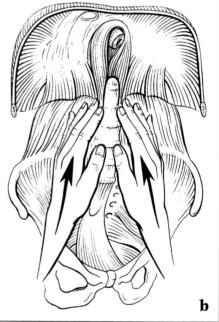

closer to the small *trochanter*. This lies at the upper end of the thigh bone, which in turn is the attachment point of the psoas. This muscle is shorter during sitting than it is when standing, and with time and our sitting habits, it isn't surprising that the psoas gets used to this length. If we get up after hours of sitting, our muscles can't adapt immediately. The result is that the iliopsoas pulls the lumbar region towards the legs, a hollow back is formed, and the pelvis tips forward. In the long run, sitting puts an enormous strain on the spine.

The liberated back

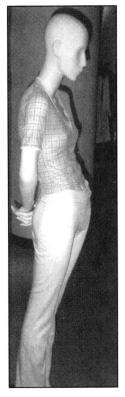

Sitting postures, stress, movement habits and lack of exercise in the western world put the curves of the spine out of balance, and thus most people have shortened hip flexor muscles (see Alternatives to stretching, page 15). In the picture at the right, you can see an example of poor posture.

As you will have noticed, it is a mannequin portraying a fashionable (but not well-aligned) portrait of a desirable ideal. If this mannequin had a voice, however, she would most likely be complaining about back pain. With the help of the picture at bottom, **a–c**, we will shortly be able to understand the problem better. We can see two boxes that are connected through a spring. The upper picture depicts the thorax, and the lower one the pelvis. Through bad posture, the spring—the lumbar spine—is badly strained (**a**). To correct this, we must enlarge the space between the boxes and stretch the compressed

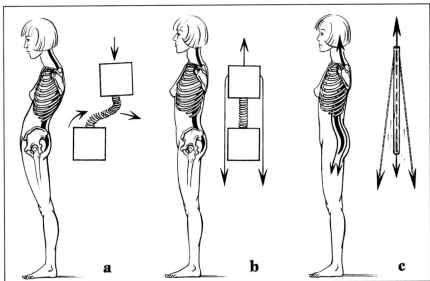

a   b   c

spring (**b**). It is not appropriate to follow the teachings of the old posture correction school by pressing against the two boxes superficially, or by forcing them with pure muscle strength. The spring has to be stretched.

The length of the lumbar region is determined by muscles that envelop the spine from all sides. The back extensors (*erector spinae* and other smaller muscles) are in the back, and in front and on the side are the iliopsoas and the *quadratus lumborum*. These are the main muscles in charge of keeping the spine erect. If one is able to learn to stretch these muscles downward, this will straighten the spine.

A comparison might help us to understand the process better. Imagine a simple tent. The tarpaulin and the towlines represent the muscles, and the tent pole is the spine. In order to put up the tent, one has to pull down on the towlines and the tarpaulin, and anchor them in the ground (**c**). If the towline and the tarpaulin are too short on one side then the tent pole (spine) will be crooked. If the pull is too weak, then the tent pole will fall down; if the pull is too strong then the tarpaulin will tear. In the following exercise, we will stretch the towlines in such a way that they are balanced and able to straighten the spine again.

Slow eccentric action for the iliopsoas

Muscles that have lost their power to straighten will not be able to fulfill their function if they are passively stretched. This means that the muscle has to participate actively in stretching. Thus we attain two goals in one exercise: the toning and the stretching of the muscles. I call this kind of stretching Slow Eccentric Action (SEA). A veritable reprogramming of the muscles has to take place for them to be able to support the spine from both sides. After SEA, many people feel a stretching of the spine as if it had been librated from a stranglehold, as the illustration opposite shows.

The following exercise, inspired by Lulu Sweigard and Bonnie Bainbridge Cohen, is very effective for solving the aforementioned problems, no matter how insignificant the exercise may seem at first. I recommend practicing it daily, especially in the evening.

1. Stand with feet pointing forward, hip-width apart, and feel the posture of your pelvis. Is the pelvis tipped forward (the front of the pelvis pointing down)? Are you standing with a hollow back?

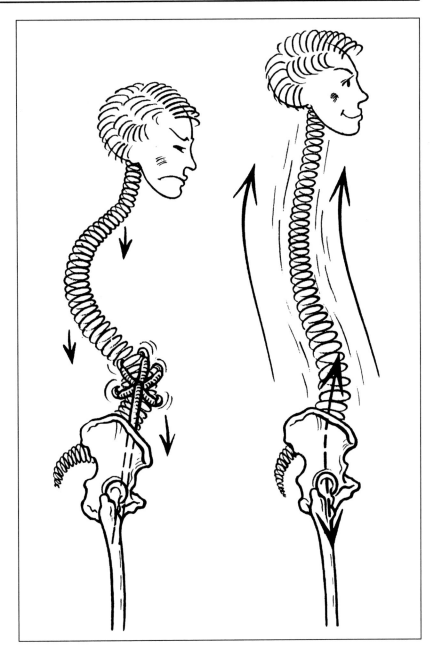

Is the pelvis tipped backward? Is the back straight? How do you have to tip the pelvis in order to have a good posture? How strongly do you have to strain your muscles to achieve this? Does the pelvis fall back into its old position as soon as you relax the muscles? If there is a mirror, look at the posture of the pelvis from the side.

2. Lie on your back in the Constructive Rest Position (see page 33), legs bent and feet on the floor. Have two Franklin balls or a rolled-up towel handy. Feel your back on the floor. Is your lumbar region lifted off the ground? Can you put your hand in between the floor and your back? Are your shoulders on the ground? Now put the two balls or the rolled up towel under the lower part of the pelvis. Keeping your knees bent, lift your feet off the ground and let your knees fall back toward your chest. The lower back will be slightly lifted off the floor where the Franklin balls are located. Don't push your back into the ground in order to correct this. It is important, however, that a hollow back doesn't develop—if it does, you can push the balls or towel further down toward your buttocks.

3. Imagine the back resting loosely like a heavy hammock. Put one hand on your belly and imagine that the organs within the pelvis and belly are soft and sinking down toward your back and the floor. Imagine the weight of the organs. To help you relax them, say inwardly: "my organs are heavy and relaxed." In the lumbar and pelvic area, next to the spine, is the iliopsoas. Imagine this muscle relaxing next to the spine.

4. Take hold of your left knee only, and slowly lower the right foot until it touches the ground. Continue to breathe with ease, and imagine that your back is hanging downward like a hammock,

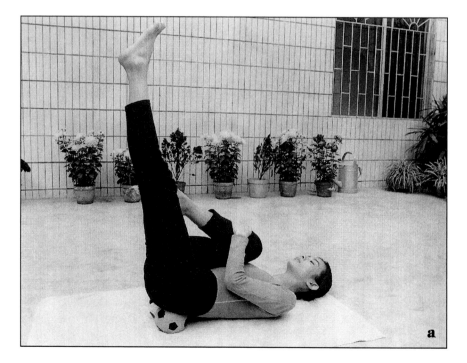

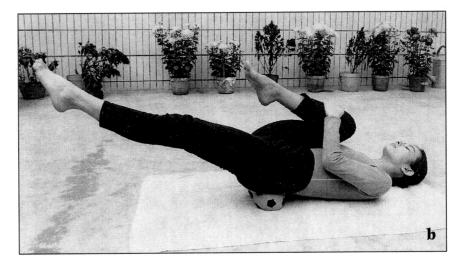

or if you prefer, like a soft, warm cat's belly. Lift the right foot back up and repeat the slow lowering action three more times.

5. Repeat the same sequence with the other leg.

6. Keep holding your right knee with your hands and stretch the left leg up in the air (see illustration **a**). Slowly lower the left leg and imagine the psoas as a river with a powerful current (**b**). Imagine the river flowing downward along the side of the spine (**c**). At the same time, imagine your back hammocking down toward the ground. Do not allow a hollow-back position to develop. The left leg should be neither twisted at the hip nor allowed drift to the side.

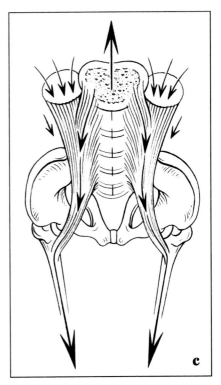

7. Lower the leg as far as is comfortable without tipping the pelvis forward and getting into a hollow-back posture. Then bend the left leg at the knee, stretch it back up in the air, and repeat the slow lowering action.

8. Repeat this movement with the left leg another five times.

Now, take the Franklin balls away and stretch both legs. Can you feel a difference between the two legs? Can you feel a difference between the right and the left side of the back? Bend the legs at the hip joint and compare the ease of movement and the amount of flexibility. You may notice that your back is more relaxed on the side of the lowered leg, and that the hip joint of the same side now feels more flexible.

9. After the exercise sequence, sit up. How easy does sitting feel? Stand up and feel what has changed in your posture. Pay special attention to your lower back; you may notice that it is more relaxed and lengthened.

10. Now, do the exercise with the right leg.

Gravity is your friend

In outer space, you can move almost effortlessly (depending on the effectiveness of your space suit, of course)! After only a week's holiday in space, however, you would most likely complain: "I feel like a ton of lead!" In everyday life, we are hardly aware of the constant pull of the earth, but gravity is constantly tugging at our every bone, muscle, tendon and organ. As we grow up, we stretch upward away from the earth. For this we need strength, flexibility and coordination. A child does not notice the exertion involved, as he or she has so much fun exploring the possibilities of movement. Many adults, however, unconsciously capitulate to the force of gravity. Slowly they slouch and sag, bones, muscles, skin and all. The good news is that this is avoidable. First, we need to change our attitudes. If we are going deal with gravity all our lives, why not make it our ally? We also breathe throughout life, there is no choice about that, so why not do it well?

To make gravity our ally, we need to understand how our body is designed. We would not be here if our bodies were not somehow structured to work with gravity. For this we turn to the opposite of gravity: the *ground reaction force*. Through conscious use of this force we can save a lot of energy, and lift our body, our face, and our spirits. A good thing about gravity is that every movement we make can be considered a workout; every movement we make exercises our postural muscles. Our daily activities support a good posture or aggravate it. It is as important to think about posture in daily life as it is during exercise. The postural improvement made during an exercise session

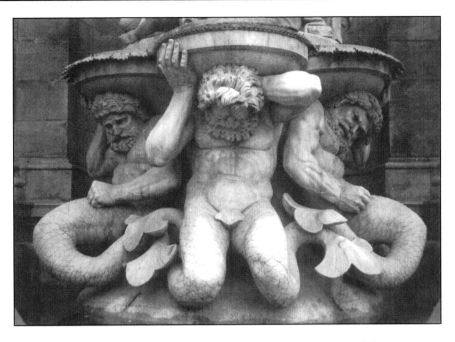

does not make up for a sagging posture during the rest of the day. Our goal is to build a lasting consciousness of our posture.

The body has two basic relationships to weight: weight is either carried from below (see illustration at the right), or pressed from above (see illustration above). The pelvic floor carries the organs; the liver and the kidneys are suspended from the diaphragm; the head sits on the atlas; and the arm hangs from the shoulder blade. If one can feel how the different structures are carried or suspended, movement coordination is improved. As we experience the interdependence of the weight of different parts of the body, we will be able to initiate movement with more awareness.

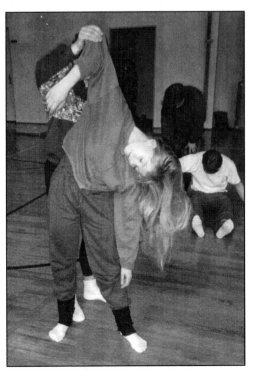

One of the best relaxation exercises for the shoulders, for example, would be to experience the weight of the shoulder girdle and the arms. This experience would automatically allow our shoulder muscles to be stretched and relaxed. The question is: why don't we do this spontaneously?

Our brain receives a constant flood of information. Body posture, temperature, speed, balance, and heart rate are constantly registered and adapted. But much of this information has to be kept from our consciousness in order for us to function at all. If we were to consciously perceive all these events, there would be a chaotic jumble of sensations in our head. When we lift a cup of coffee, for example, we don't feel the weight of the arm, we simply feel the cup. The arm feels as light as a feather, even though the arm is quite a bit heavier than the cup (see illustration **a**). If we habitually pull our shoulders

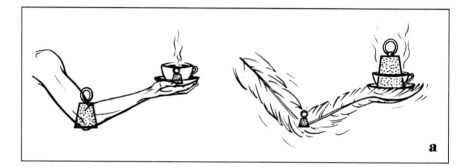

a

up against gravity, the body does not send the information to our brain constantly. This would simply drive us crazy. The brain shuts off the sensation for the time being, so that we can function. Eventually we become aware of tension. We have been holding our shoulders up against gravity for a while now and it will take a bit of awareness to change the situation.

The key to change is, therefore, becoming aware of what our bodies are doing. This means focusing on the position of our shoulders, practicing better posture and alignment, embracing a new position, and

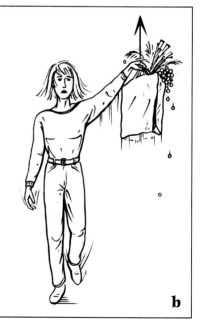

b

maintaining it in daily life [picking up shopping bags with relaxed shoulders, for example (**b**)].

Sand flows from the shoulders

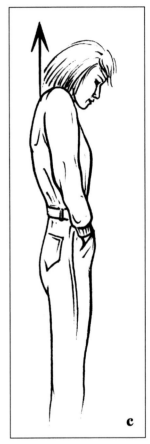

1. First ask yourself: what is weight? What is my concept of weight? Of suspension?

2. Lift your shoulders up and then let them fall while breathing out. Try to feel the weight of your shoulders and arms. Lift the shoulders up again and let them sink back down in slow motion. Think: "my shoulders are relaxed and heavy."

3. Let your shoulders hang in a relaxed way, without letting the spine slump.

4. Imagine that your shoulders and arms are filled with sand. Lift your shoulders up. While lowering them, imagine that the sand is flowing out of your shoulders from the seams between the arms and shoulders, from the elbows and from the finger tips (**c**).

5. Repeat the lowering of the shoulders once more with the image of the sand flowing from the shoulders' seams, the elbows and the fingers.

6. Lift and lower your shoulders twice more with a "Haaah" sound as you do this.

c

Tapping the shoulders

For this exercise you will need a partner and two Franklin balls. Stand behind your partner and hold the two balls loosely in your hands. Tap the shoulders of your partner gently with the balls. Slowly move the balls outward toward the arms and downward toward the hands while continuing to tap. Repeat this gentle tapping in the same direction two or three times. Meanwhile, your partner imagines that each single cell in the shoulders is being tapped. Each cell is relaxed, like thousands of fluffed-up tiny cushions. By letting go of shoulder tension you may start to feel your base: the pelvis, legs, and feet.

The sound of good posture

We know that music that can have a healing effect on us, but so can the sounds we can make ourselves. One doesn't have to be able to sing well; simple sounds like "Aaaaa," vocalized with an open mouth, or "Mmm," hummed with a closed mouth, can have an astonishing effect. The ancient Egyptians are said to have used the power of the voice therapeutically.

Lifting the breastbone

Many people have a slightly caved-in chest and hunched shoulders. This posture is disadvantageous to the whole body (see photograph, page 61).

The heart, located behind the breastbone, is pressured and the lungs cannot fully expand. Try this exercise:

1. In a standing position gently tap your breastbone.

2. Put your hand flat on the breastbone and start to make a few "Aaaaa" sounds with an open mouth. You will probably feel the breastbone vibrating gently.

3. Try to vary the pitch in such a way that the breastbone vibrates at different frequencies.

4. Like finding the right radio station, look for the pitch that makes the breastbone vibrate the most.

5. Continue to make sounds for two or three minutes.

6. Focus on the lower as well as the upper part of the breastbone.

7. Imagine that you are able to make your heart, which lies a little to the left behind the lower part of the breastbone, vibrate as well.

8. Again, like tuning into a radio station, try to find the pitch that vibrates the heart.

9. Continue as long as it feels comfortable and enjoyable, alternating between vibrating the breastbone and the heart.

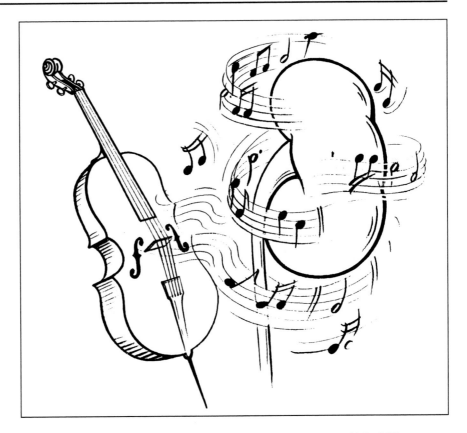

10. After finishing the exercise, ask yourself: "do I still feel like slumping into a bad posture?"

The coccyx

For a rocket to take off into space, a downward thrust is needed. This is also true for the spine: for it to straighten, a certain downward thrust is necessary. In this context, special attention should be paid to the coccyx, the lowest part of the spine. The thrust of the spine is produced here, as the coccyx is connected to the pelvic floor, the muscular base of the upper body.

Unfortunately the coccyx is often considered a superfluous remnant of mankind's dim and distant past. This is far from being true—without the cooperation of the coccyx and the activation of the pelvic floor connected to it, the spine and our entire body posture would be at risk. At a particular point in our embryonic development, the coccyx is as long as the rest of our body. In many animals, the coccyx stays long and becomes the tail. It serves to balance the body during jumps and turns, and also for communication, as well as for getting rid of annoying insects! We humans don't have to worry so much about insects, but the muscles that used to move the tail remain as important pelvic floor muscles. The tail muscles have been moved forward to connect to and support the organs of the pelvis. The activation of the coccyx is therefore an obvious way of strengthening those muscles. Furthermore, the coccyx plays an important role in human posture and balance.

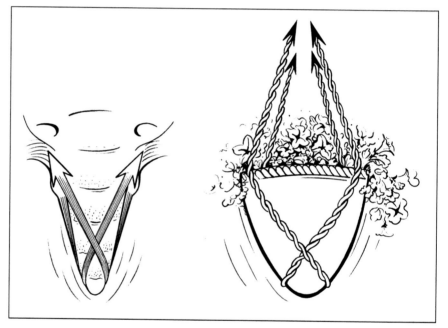

In the illustration above, we can see the coccyx surrounded by ligaments, like a hanging flowerpot. The ligaments are the lower end of the long chain that is responsible for the anchoring of the spine and the conservation of a three-dimensional form under constant flux. The coccyx is a combination of elastic ligaments, muscles, and space-maintaining struts (the bones). This ingenious system can become unbalanced by a lack of movement, as well as by insufficient anchoring of the coccyx in the pelvic floor.

Exercise: the moving coccyx

1. Lying on your back, put a Franklin ball under the coccyx and one under your head, and feel the upper and lower ends of the spine.

2. Start to move the coccyx. You can move it up and down, left and right, and rotate it. Explore all the possible movements of the coccyx. As you also have a ball under your head, it is possible to observe how the movements of the coccyx and the head are connected.

3. Stand up and touch your coccyx with one hand. Stand with feet wide apart. Try to swing the coccyx left and right. At first, you will think it impossible, but try nevertheless. You can imagine that the coccyx used to be long enough to brush against the ground while swinging.

4. You can also imagine that the coccyx is a silk band moving through space (see illustration below).

5. Swing the coccyx to the front and back. As you swing to the front, feel the coccyx moving closer to the front of the pelvis and the pubic bone. As you swing to the back, feel it moving further away from the pubic bone.

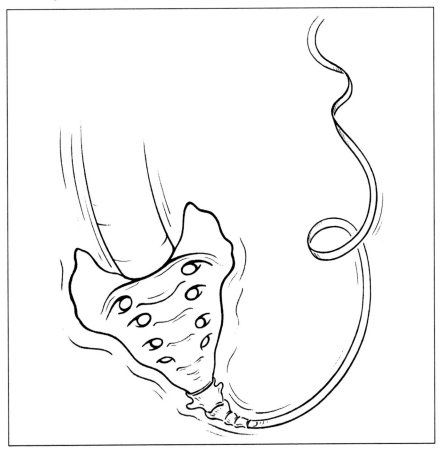

6. Bring your feet together in a parallel position, and feel what has changed in your posture.

Experience: the bouncing coccyx

Once I was going for a walk, thinking about my coccyx (admittedly not one's usual thoughts during a walk), when I noticed a bird flying above me. I saw that it was fanning out its tail feathers and then pressing its wings against its body. I took this as an inspiration for my coccyx. I imagined my coccyx as a feathered tail, fanned it out and closed it again; I added my breath to the image. While inhaling, I let the feathers widen, and while exhaling I closed them again. The effect of this image was that my gait became looser and the hip joints freer. I thanked the bird and saw once more that we are surrounded by the most diverse sources of inspiration for the improved functioning of our bodies.

5 Discovering the Organs

Because of the current style of exercising, oriented toward the development of muscle, we are no longer aware of the part our organs play in movement and posture. They do, in fact, play an important role in the efficient execution of sport, gymnastics and the movements of daily life. Organs are by their nature the core weight of our body; they are nourishing, soft and elastic. After a hearty meal we can feel the quality of the organs, their heaviness and their increased size. Likewise, when we are tired, we withdraw into the "organ state," preferably into a soft, warm bed where we feel like a protected baby. Babies are often in the organ state, because their organs dominate their limbs in size and capability. A baby's liver, for example, is huge in relation to the rest of its body. As adults, the pressure to perform and the pace of daily life may deplete the organs. We don't feel when it is time to let the organs rest, nor do we know how to exercise them as we do our muscles. One of our goals, therefore, should be to balance the inner and outer activities of the body. Let us now become conscious of our organs and find out how such awareness can support us in our daily life.

The organs, the skeleton, and the muscular system

Problems which manifest themselves in the muscular system or in the joints have their origin in unfavorable organ positions or movements. Again and again I see people tensing and putting pressure on their organs during exercise. Discovering the organs not only relieves the whole movement apparatus of much of its load, but also improves metabolism and digestion; eventually we begin to feel the relationship between the functioning of the organs and our daily movement and exercise.

Figuratively speaking, the organs live in the skeleton. Like good inhabitants, they should not be a burden but be a support to their host, and should contribute to the upkeep of their dwelling. We can compare the skeleton to a frame and the organs to a large balloon. Looking at the figures on page 76, we can see **a**, the skeleton without

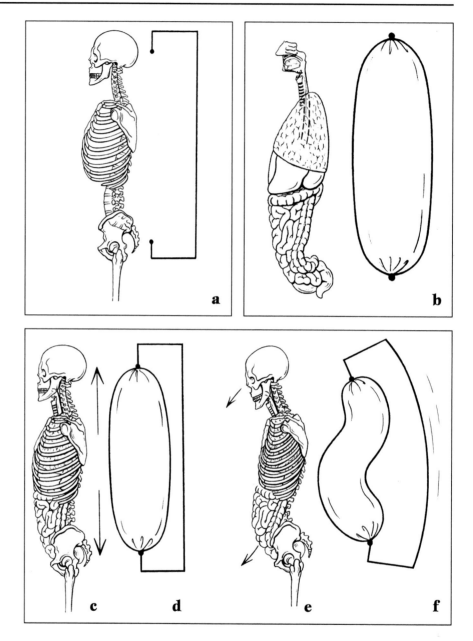

organs, and **b**, the organs without the skeleton. These two systems are dependent on each other to function properly. On one hand, the organs hang onto the skeleton in figure **c**. On the other, the force and elasticity of the organs support the posture of the skeleton in figure **d**.

A water-filled balloon is not dissimilar to an organ in its consistency.

When we hold such a balloon gently between two fingers, we can feel that it fills the space between the fingers in an elastic sort of way. The balloon can carry weight and at the same time fill space with outward pressure. If the balloon is slack (**f**), then the space between the fingers lessens. The human body is similar. In figure **c** we can see a harmonious balance between the organs and the skeleton. Figure **e**, in contrast, shows slack organs and their effect on the posture of the body.

The colon, pelvis, and pelvic base

The interdependence of the organs and the skeleton can be seen when looking in detail: the rectum and anus, for example, are attached to the pelvic bone by muscles and connective tissues. The base of the pelvis acts as a kind of trampoline that is attached all around the pelvic bone and the coccyx; organs, muscles and bones in this area are directly dependent on each other for their correct functioning. Flatulence and digestive problems lead to either tension or slackness in nearby muscles; these problems are then passed on to the bones and joints. The spine and the adjacent joints of the ilium and the sacrum also suffer, and thus the hip joint comes under increased pressure.

Organ movement

What is meant by *organ movement*? Most of the time we are not aware of this movement, even though it is taking place all the time. *Peristalsis*, a rhythmic contraction of the intestines, is a well-known organ movement that takes care of transporting food throughout the body.

But other organs move as well. The kidney, for example, is attached to the diaphragm by connective tissue. Because the diaphragm moves downwards when we inhale, the kidney moves down as well. When we exhale, the diaphragm moves up, and so does the kidney. Every time we breathe, the kidney glides like a sleigh through snow, and is moved by the diaphragm. At an average breathing rate, a kidney moves over three hundred yards a day. If the kidney is not moving properly, due to poor breathing, posture or digestive problems can lead to back pain. Exercises involving muscle relaxation are only a temporary aid, since the problem lies in the movement of the organ.

In my classes, I discover again and again that participants can't picture their organs. They can imagine only an empty space, a black hole, where their organs are. A simple and useful example of an image of the organs is that of elastic balloons arranged in layers. It is important to fill in this imaginary empty space, so that you may feel the satisfying and relaxing sensation of your organs.

Hot water bottle on the belly

Fill a hot water bottle with warm water and get comfortable in the Constructive Rest Position (see page 33). Put the hot water bottle on the belly, but take care that it is not too heavy and at a comfortable temperature. You'll feel immediately a pleasant warmth seeping into your belly, radiating out to all the organs.

Again imagine the organs as water-filled balloons. Up to the right under the ribs is the liver, and behind it the right kidney. To the left is the stomach, and behind that, the left kidney and the spleen. In the direction of the belly button, under these organs, is the transverse colon, and further down toward the pelvis is the small intestine. The rising colon lies to the right, and then descending to the left, the small intestine. The bladder can be found right under the pubic bone. Move the hot water bottle to different areas of the belly. Imagine that the organs are filling up with a warm feeling, and let them take up their rightful place in your body awareness.

Breathing and the organs

Each breath massages the organs between the moving belly muscles and the diaphragm. While breathing in, the diaphragm lowers and pushes the organs downward. As the organs can't move to the back because they meet the spine, they move forward and are caught, as if in a hammock, by the expanding belly muscles (illustration **a**). The pelvic floor is also part of this elastic cushioning system, and functions like a slow-motion trampoline which receives the organs during inhalation, and during exhalation helps to push them upward again (see also Chapter 6, Breathing). The belly muscle hammock pushes the organs gently back during exhalation, and they glide upward as if on a slide, and help the diaphragm to relax. The diaphragm is not quite passive during this activity, but helps the lifting action like a suction device (illustration **b**). Breathing is important to the maintenance of flexible and supple organs.

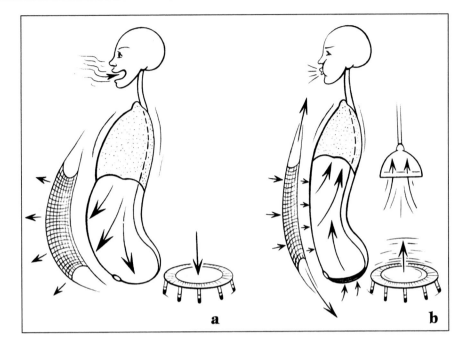

a   b

Lying on air-filled balls

For work with the organs, large, soft, air-filled balls are especially useful as they are more elastic than the customary sitting balls, and they adapt to the body. For the following exercise it is ideal have a large and a small ball at hand, but you may use a large and a small cushion.

1. Lie on your stomach. Put the large ball (or cushion) under the belly, and the small one under the breastbone (see illustration).

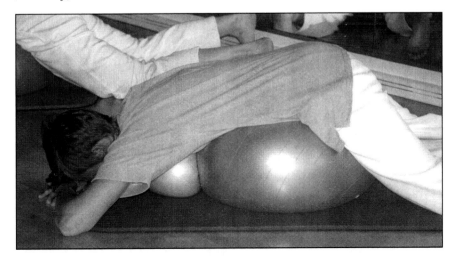

2. Let yourself sink into the balls. Feel the heaviness of the organs, and transfer their weight to the balls.

3. Mentally direct your breathing into the different organs. Visualize your breath flowing around the organs, surrounding them with a soft, cozy feeling.

4. Feel the rocking of the organs between the belly muscles and the diaphragm.

5. When you breathe in, visualize the diaphragm lowering and pushing the organs down. When you breathe out, feel the belly muscles lifting the organs gently upward.

6. Stay in this position for about fifteen minutes (longer if it feels good).

7. After standing up, notice any changes. You may well feel very tired and heavy; perhaps you need to slow down a little. Once we start to become acquainted with the organ state, this is a very natural reaction.

Organs on the slide

1. Before starting this exercise, focus on the position of your organs while standing up. Do they feel as if they are pulling the pelvis or spine forward? Do they feel well supported by the pelvic floor and abdominal muscles?

2. Lie down in the Constructive Rest Position and imagine your abdominal organs. Visualize the organs resting on the spine and the back of your body.

3. Visualize the dome of the diaphragm and the organs resting within it (the spleen, kidneys, stomach, pancreas, and liver). The diaphragm arches protectively around these organs.

4. Now lift the pelvis upward. Start this movement at the very bottom end of the spine, with the tail bone (coccyx).

5. When the pelvis is lifted so that your back is slanted down toward the shoulders, imagine all the organs sliding down and resting on the diaphragm.

6. Repeat the exercise a few times. Stand up slowly and feel what has changed in the position of your organs and in your posture. You may notice a release of tension in your lower back.

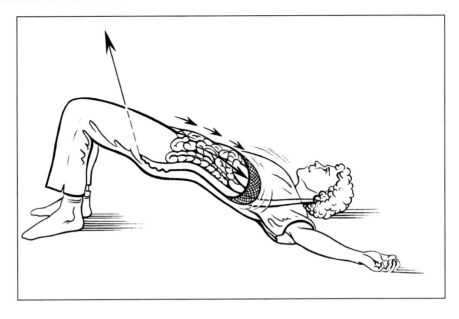

The mesentery

Muscles, ligaments and connective tissue often act as mediator between the skeleton and the organs. An important example of this relationship is the *mesentery*. The mesentery uses connective tissue to connect the intestines to the back of the abdominal wall, which lies on the spine. It folds around the intestines and holds them in alignment (see illustration). It is thus obvious that the state of the intestines is reflected in the musculature of the back. Slack and bloated organs tend to pull the spine forward and produce a hyper-extended (hollowed) spine and lower back tension.

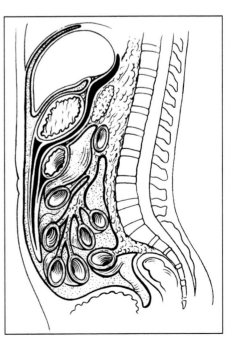

Lie down in the CRP (see page 33), and picture the following: the mesentery is like a beautiful ocean plant anchored on the ocean floor with tiny floating leaves. The spine represents the ground of the ocean and the mesentery and intestines the plant with its floating whorls.

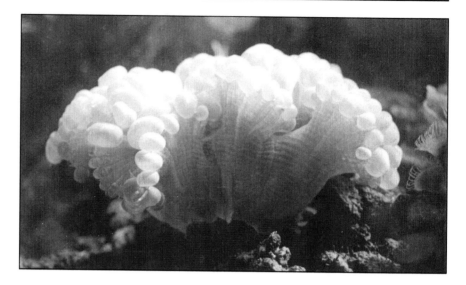

The spine moves the intestines

Lying on the air-filled balls, visualize the following situation, which you may well have experienced. Underwater your hair floats softly around your head. The spine can move the mesentery just as the movement of your head can make your hair float gently around your head in the water. Move your spine, and try to be aware that with each movement of the spine, the intestines will also move. Stand up. Move your spine and visualize the mesentery and the intestines being swung back and forth. Imagine that you are pulling them in toward the spine, like a fisherman pulling in nets, in order to relieve the spine and maintain good posture.

The kidney

The right kidney lies behind the liver on the right *psoas* muscle, and the left kidney lies behind the stomach on the left psoas muscle. The kidney is kept loosely in position by the suction effect of the diaphragm and a connective tissue pouch, and through the pressure of the stomach and other muscles. This allows the kidney an amazing amount of flexibility. The kidney has a great influence on the state of the sacroiliac articulation, the knee, the lumbar region and the back in general. Workshop participants often report mental clarity and relaxation of the back after the exercise that follows.

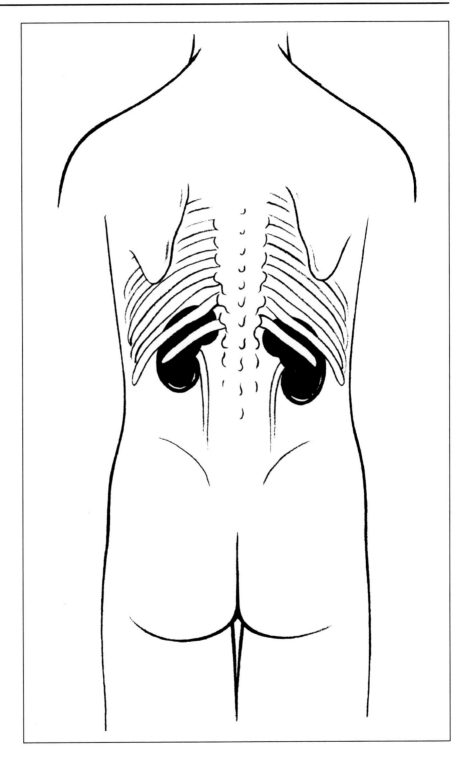

Kidney breathing

1. In a sitting position, touch your kidneys with both your hands at the mid-level of your back.

2. Guide your breathing into the kidneys. Imagine that your kidneys are doing the breathing.

3. Exhale with an "Sss" sound, and imagine the kidneys relaxing. This way, they'll be better able to fill out their allotted space. (You know the feeling—when you are relaxed, you tend to take up more space.)

4. After a few minutes take your hands away and feel your kidneys. How do your back and posture feel? Has your breathing pattern changed? Also notice changes in standing and walking.

5. Now do a few knee bends. Imagine the kidneys being carried up and down.

6. Imagine that the strength of the legs is transferred to the kidneys, as if the legs were in direct contact with the kidneys. Exercise for a few minutes until you feel that your kidneys are supported by your legs. Go for a walk and make note of any changes.

The bladder

The bladder is located behind the pubic bone. When it is full, it can be felt just above the pubic bone. Behind and above the female bladder we find the uterus; in men the lowest part of the small intestine is located here. Beneath the male bladder we find the prostate. The bladder is supported by pelvic floor musculature as well as an array of ligaments.

From the kidney to the bladder

1. While resting on the floor, put your hands on your bladder and see if you can feel it move as you breathe in and out.

2. Imagine the two kidneys and the bladder forming the corners of a triangle. Imagine this triangle slightly increasing in size when you inhale, and slightly decreasing in size when you exhale.

3. Compare the orientation of the triangle with the floor beneath

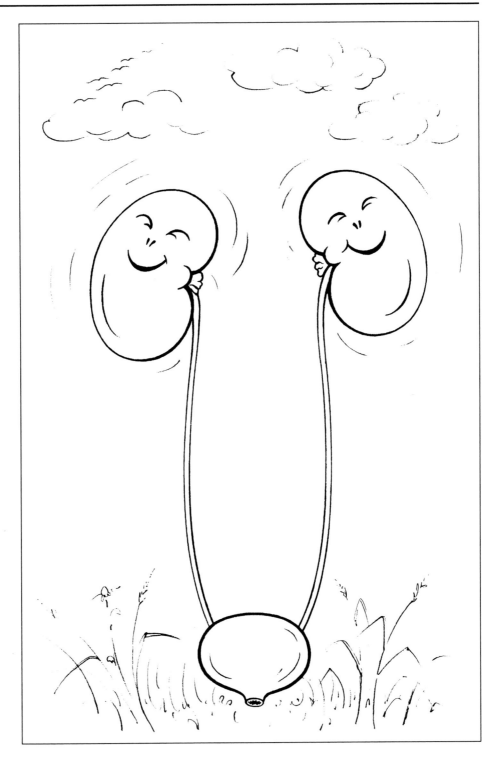

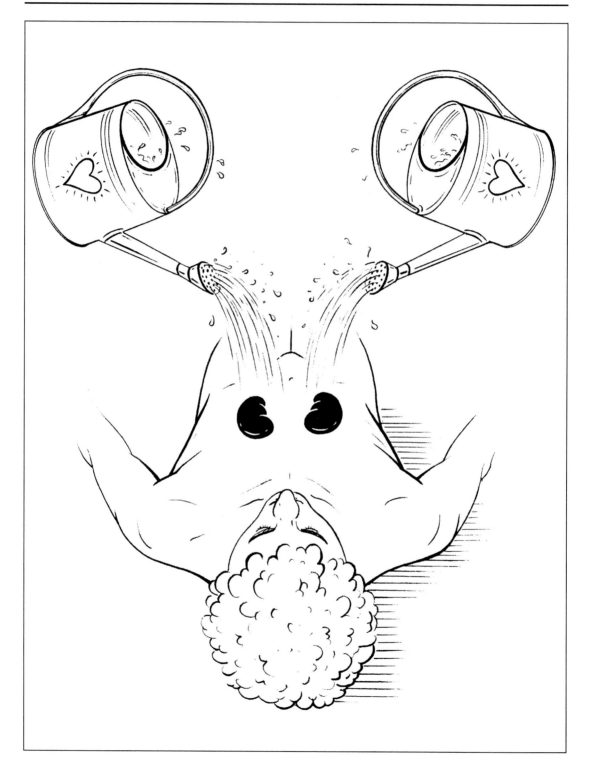

you. Is one of the corners lower than the others? Is one of the sides of the triangle longer than the others?

4. Image the two *urethras*, the tubes connecting the kidney to the bladder; they lie on the psoas muscle. Imagine that you are able to send your breath from the kidneys through the urethrae into the bladder. You may even make an "Aah" sound as you imagine this.

5. Take your time to get up off the floor and feel what has changed in your posture.

6. Standing, visualize the kidneys and the bladder. Imagine the kidneys floating upward like little balloons, while the bladder is anchored in the pelvis.

Musical kidneys

Play some of your favorite music. Imagine the music wrapping itself around your kidneys, protecting and caring for them. The music gives your kidneys great joy and makes them happy. They want to dance to the music! Try initiating some movement from the kidneys, even if this sounds strange at first.

Refreshing the kidneys

Visualize the kidneys being recharged, nourished and fuelled with fresh energy. Imagine "kidney water" flushing and regenerating the kidneys.

The heart and the lungs

Our posture greatly affects the position and level of tension of the heart. The heart lies on the left behind the breastbone and sandwiched by the lungs. It sits on the diaphragm and is tied to it by connective tissue. This is why the heart rides up and down on the diaphragm with each breath you take (as in the illustration on the following page). During inhalation, the diaphragm moves down and pulls the bottom of the heart with it. As the heart is also attached at the top, it receives a bit of a stretch.

Each breath is thus massaging the heart. Slack and shallow breathing minimizes the built-in therapeutic effect. If the upper body is

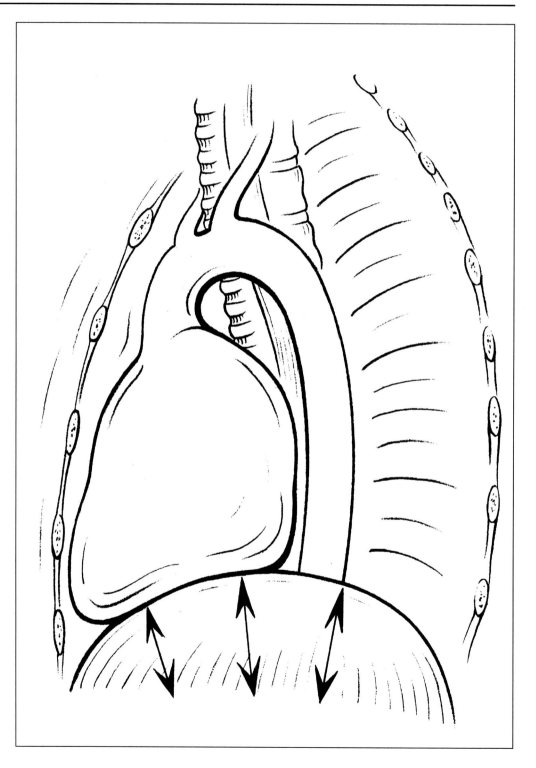

slouched, the heart is compressed by the breastbone, diaphragm and lungs, whereas good posture relieves the heart of excess pressure.

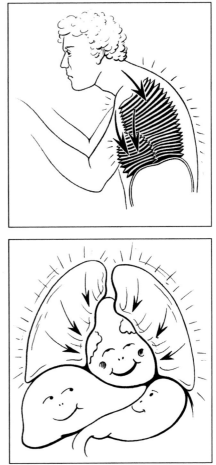

The lungs are a kind of air sponge; instead of soaking up water, they soak up air. If the windpipe is included in the image, then this sponge has the form of a tree standing on its head. Its task is to guide as much air as possible into its tiny, winding branches, and to let oxygen pass through its extremely thin walls into the body. The right lung is larger than the left, and has three *lobes* (see illustration on the following page). The left lung has only two lobes, as the heart has to share its space with them.

As already mentioned, the lungs, like any other organ, contribute to our flexibility, posture and vital inner volume. The lungs fill out the thorax. Inflexible lungs impede the movement of the shoulder girdle and the thorax. In addition, an inflexible thorax prevents coordinated arm movement. If the lungs are constantly pushed down through a slouched upper body posture, the tightening can become permanent and can restrict our overall breathing capacity. It is important to decompress the lungs so that they take up their full space and use their volume optimally to supply our cells with oxygen. This is a prime rejuvenating practice for our body.

Liberating the lungs

1. Sit down at a table with a Franklin ball handy.

2. Put your right forearm on the ball. Move your arm by rolling it on the ball.

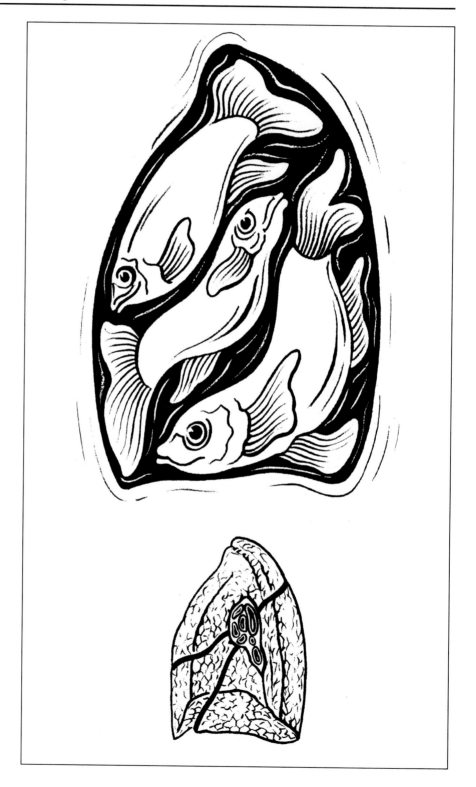

3. Try different movements that feel good to you: stretch out your arm, pull it back, rotate it inward and outward.

4. Feel the movement of the shoulder blade. Many muscles are attached to the shoulder blade, and the balanced functioning of these muscles is very important for the entire shoulder. A movement of the arm often means a movement of the shoulder blade as well. Practice initiating the movements of the arm with the shoulder blade.

5. Imagine that you can move the lungs elastically, just as if they were twisting and turning, moving your arm on the ball.

6. Imagine the lobes of the lungs sliding on top of each other, like slippery fish, bars of soap or wet sponges.

7. Imagine your movement aiding the ventilation of the lungs.

8. Now take a moment to compare the length and flexibility of both your arms. Maybe you can feel that the right arm has become longer than the left one. Perhaps the whole shoulder is more relaxed. Can you feel that your right lung fills more easily with air? Does the lung on the right feel more lifted?

9. Repeat the exercise on your left side.

Lifting the heart

This exercise is for happiness; it invigorates the mind and activates the circulation. Hold your hands in loose fists on your breastbone, knuckles pointing towards each other, and your thumbs lying on your ribs. Slowly breathe in and stroke your hands upward along your breastbone, turning your fists and forearms outward. Imagine that your heart is floating upward. Slowly look up to the ceiling (or, even better, the sky), while fanning out your fingers and pointing them upward.

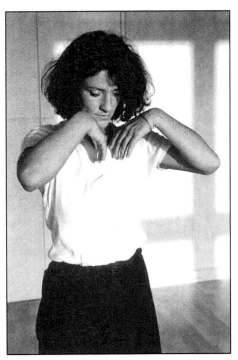

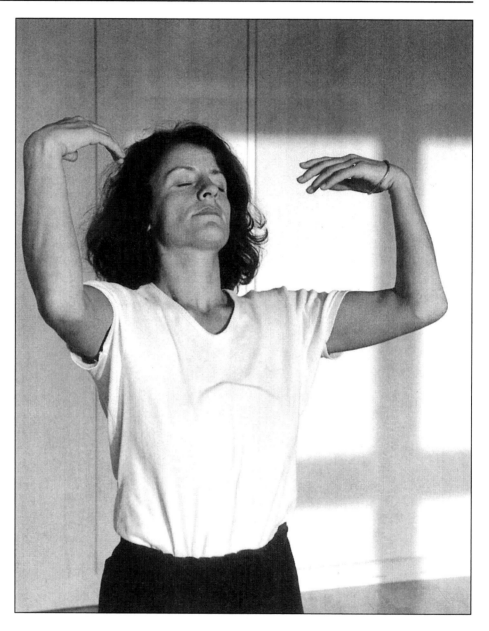

While breathing out, do the same hand movements the other way around. Close your fingers into a fist and stroke downward over your breastbone.

Repeat the lifting and lowering of the heart three times. The third time, leave your heart up (in your imagination) while you lower your arms and your head. How does it feel to walk around with a lifted heart? Medicine for the soul!

The miracle of the intelligent cell

The cell is a self-contained living unit with its own life plan and certain specific tasks. Each cell in our body is very intelligent and self-sacrificing. I purposefully choose the term "intelligent" to describe how the many functions that a cell performs show an inner knowledge that surpasses any current bio-chemical explanation. Many cells are even prepared to die for the good of the whole, and without such inner cell sacrifices, the human body would not survive.

A two-layered skin surrounds each cell: the *plasma membrane*. This membrane is constantly shifting and changing shape. The changing around of molecules within this membrane is even referred to by the term "flip-flop phenomenon." Some cells move about with the help of leg-like protrusions that they create on the spot when needed. Thus they can pull themselves forward, crawl, and make rolling and turning movements. It is quite miraculous that something as small and complex as a cell, which we are still far from understanding entirely, can function so perfectly.

If we are looking for the cause of an illness, we often forget that the situation has most often developed over a long period of time due to our own behavior. Simply changing our diet is not enough; we have to change our attitude toward our body, right down to the cellular level. A human being is a community of cells that performs best with our conscious support.

Cell voyager

Lie down in the CRP (see page 33) and imagine a single cell of your body. Visualize the cell membrane, the plasma and the *organelles* (mini-organs of the cell). Enter this cell in your imagination and go on a journey of discovery.

First, wander through the space between the outer and inner cell membrane. This is the area where there is an intense exchange of information. The outer membrane is directed towards the extra-cellular world. Within each cell is lively and intelligent activity. Harmful substances are turned into harmless ones, and energy is gained from the simplest components. Vital hormones and proteins are produced here.

Take an imaginary swim between the organelles. Next to you, *mito-chondria* are producing energy; *ribosomes* are masters at producing proteins. In front of you an Eiffel Tower-like structure is being put together, and on the other side of the cell, with similar speed, a small Golden Gate bridge is taken apart; the *microtubule*, your mobile cell construction unit, is at work. Imagine that your movements also move the cell organelles. Push an organelle with your hand and it floats away like a raft on water. Breathe in and feel how inhalation is happening all around you. Exhale and feel a breeze of movement touching the organelles.

Return from your cellular journey. Are you surprised at the masterful capacities of your cells, which have taken care of all these functions without your knowing? Promise your cells to do something good for them today and every day. Fulfilling this promise is only a thought away.

6 Breathing

We breathe throughout our lives. Why not be good at it? Breathing is vital to provide energy and to regenerate our bodies. It is a permanent and vital process that connects us intimately with the air that surrounds us. We hardly ever think about the fact that our connection with the air is more important than our connection with our arms. We can live without an arm but not without air. We are constantly busy assimilating and expelling part of our surroundings—the air.

For oxygen to enter the bloodstream, the air meets the *alveoli*—baglike end points in the lungs with a surface of over one hundred square yards. Breathing is the most intimate exchange between our inner and outer worlds. Thousands of cubic yards of air travel through us in a lifetime. If someone smokes in your surrounding area, you could say that they are sending a destructive chemical via the air directly into your body. Smoke influences the organs of the smoker in the most direct sense and thus also the cells of fellow human beings.

Breathing needs space

In order for us to breathe, the inner volume of the lungs needs to expand. Without this expansion, and the resulting suction effect, no air can enter. A whole row of muscles, bones and organs takes care of this three-dimensional expansion with complex teamwork at the level of a symphony orchestra.

The diaphragm is rightly called the central breathing muscle, and when it comes to bones, the ribs have the key position. Let's have a look at the breathing process in a simplified form. The diaphragm is a dome-shaped structure that moves the floor of the airtight lungs downward, expanding them and creating negative pressure, sucking air into the lungs. This is the contraction phase of the diaphragm. Another dome at the base of the spine is formed by the pelvic floor, which is connected via the frontal longitudinal ligament to the diaphragm (see illustration). The organs of the belly and the pelvis are packed in between these two domes.

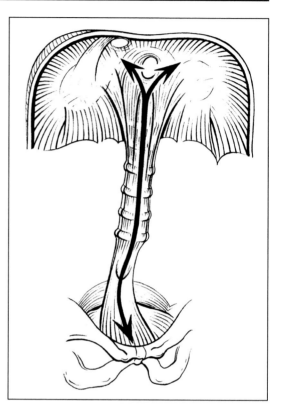

The diaphragm lies on the liver, the kidneys and the stomach, so that breathing directly massages these organs and indirectly massages others. During inhalation the belly widens to make space for the organs, and even the pelvic floor does its part and stretches as much as it can. The stomach and pelvic floor muscles work together and are the tension counterparts of the diaphragm (see also page 97). The spine also stretches slightly during inhalation, and it, too, creates more space for breathing. The ribs widen sideways and upward, to the front and back, and thus provide additional expansion of the lungs. Often one expands the thorax primarily to the front, which may cause tension in the back. It is important to feel the expansion of the ribs as a three-dimensional event.

The uppermost tips of the lungs reach the shoulder area. During inhalation, they can even move into the upper rib area. Unfortunately, tense and slumped shoulders often block this path. I would like to emphasize that deep breathing doesn't rely on abdominal breathing alone, but on the flexibility of all structures involved. The goal is to create an elastic container for the lungs and all the necessary possibilities of expansion.

During exhalation, the dome of the diaphragm rises. To allow this, the fibers of the diaphragm have to stretch. I have discovered that many people find this difficult to comprehend. How can the dome rise when the diaphragm relaxes? The diaphragm has a considerable back-up system, the stomach muscles and the pelvic floor, which actively support exhalation. They contract and push the organs back up towards the diaphragm. They are not able to do this without the help of the diaphragm, which, when it arches upward, creates suction that pulls the organs with it.

Tensing as a slimming strategy

Sucking in the belly muscles as a posture and slimming strategy has marked disadvantages. Breathing is blocked; if one wants to inhale, the stomach muscles and the pelvic floor have to let go. This is not possible with tensed abdominals, because a permanent tensing of the diaphragm will ensue, a state in which many people spend a large part of their lives. In this state the world never looks very friendly; you are never able to let go, and it seems as if everything is against you, even your own diaphragm! Stress and back pain are the natural consequences; the ribs stay in a lifted position and cannot fall back properly in relation to the body's axis, tightening the back muscles as well.

Breathing and the stomach muscles

In this exercise, we will experience the effect of the stomach muscles on breathing: pull your stomach way in and make your waist thin. Now try to breathe in. It's simply impossible. To sum up, the best training for the stomach muscles is relaxed breathing, as they are exercised with each breath.

The movement of the diaphragm

Practice this exercise while sitting: during inhalation the diaphragm moves down and the ribs widen. As you inhale, imagine that your diaphragm is floating down softly and effortlessly, like a piece of silk. Let this piece of silk float down as loosely and gently as possible, coming to rest on your abdominal organs. As you exhale, imagine that this cloth is carried up again with the organs. To deepen the exhalation, imagine the fibers of your diaphragm stretching. Put your hands on both sides of the lower ribs. As you breathe out, imagine the dome of your diaphragm floating up as high as possible and withdrawing from your hands, which move with the ribs toward the center of the body. During this exercise it is very important to breathe normally; don't make a special effort to breathe deeply.

The movement of the ribs

Sit down in such a way that you balance on your sit bones, and don't lean back on your chair. Touch your breastbone and glide your fingers to the lower end of the breastbone. This spot is called the *xyphoid process* of the breastbone. It should be soft to make deep breathing possible, and elastic like rubber. With the fingers of both hands, follow the descending edges of your ribs toward your back: you should feel a soft, bouncy sensation. Imagine that your ribs swing out like an apron of pleats (see illustration).

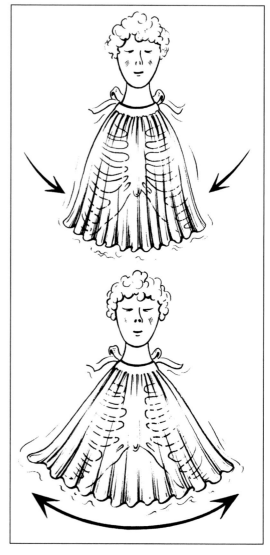

See the pleats widening. During inhalation, let the apron fall back again toward the center axis of the body. The ribs swing as loosely as possible, in and out, like soft material. In order to make the xyphoid process more flexible, imagine that it is swinging back and forth like a flag in the wind while you breathe in and out (see illustration).

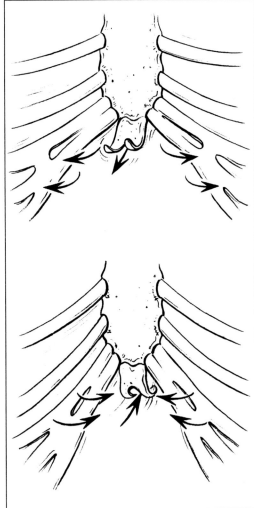

Breathing takes place inside the cells

The lungs are in some sense just a means to an end, as the actual breathing process takes place inside the cells. Oxygen, which has been guided in a complex fashion into the body, is first used here. A cell that can't breathe will die. Breathing takes place in the entire body, not just in the lungs. The following exercises will help to convey this:

Whole body breathing (1)

1. Observe your breathing lying down in the CRP with your arms next to your body on the floor. Where in the body can you feel your breathing? Do you feel it in your thorax? In the belly? Maybe in the shoulders? In the spine? Perhaps in the arms and legs? Does your breath create movement in your body? Where do you feel this movement?

2. Imagine that you are able to guide your breathing into your right arm. Imagine the right arm to be spacious like the inside of a balloon. Breathe into the entire right arm all the way to the tips of your fingers. Exhale out of your right arm completely.

3. It now feels as if the wish to breathe is actually coming from the right arm. We are breathing because the right arm wants to breathe.

4. After a few minutes, notice your left arm. How does the left arm feel in comparison to the right "breathing" arm? Heavier? Lighter? Larger? Smaller?

5. Now breathe into the left arm. The left arm is almost able to breathe, in and out, as if the wish to breathe was coming from it.

6. Repeat the same process with the right and left leg.

7. Now imagine that the entire body is breathing. Experience breathing as something which is caused by the entire body, almost as if it were a single huge lung. Maybe there are still places that are without breath. Don't worry; perhaps the next breath will find its way there as well.

Whole body breathing (2)

1. Lie down again in the CRP and observe your breathing. Let the breathing just happen; you're an observer who doesn't interfere with what is happening.

2. Feel the large surface of the inside of your lungs, which contains five hundred million alveoli. Imagine that this entire surface is able to absorb oxygen. All is calm here, and oxygen can enter the bloodstream without any effort at all.

3. Observe your skin. Imagine that your skin is a huge breathing organ; each pore of the skin is able to breathe. Feel how you are surrounded by air, a never-ending source of oxygen.

4. Remember that a membrane surrounds the cells, and that this also breathes. Your body is a community of breathing cells.

5. The cells breathe with the same calm as the lungs. Oxygen is supplied, the cells breathe in, and the cells breathe out.

6. Return to whole body breathing and feel the individual cells and the lungs breathing at the same time.

7. Give yourself plenty of time to wake up from this experience, and then stand up again. Can you feel whole body breathing while standing up?

Playful blood cells

Oxygen is supplied to the body entirely by the red blood cells. They look like plates with very broad, round edges. Imagine the red blood cells absorbing oxygen in the lungs and effortlessly carrying their precious freight to all the cells of the body. No cell is left out. Oxygen is distributed to all corners of the body. If you sense a place in your body that feels neglected or cramped, provide it with extra red blood cells. They flit and sway playfully through your arteries, doing their work with vigor. No capillary vessel is too small for them, no place in the body too remote or insignificant.

Laughing to breathe

Would you be surprised to learn that laughing improves your breathing? Laughing relaxes the breathing muscles and tones the tissues in a perfectly natural way. Learning to laugh is an important part of my classes, even though many participants have difficulty accepting that such an ordinary activity can be so beneficial. A common question from participants in these workshops is "when are we going to do 'proper' breathing exercises?" People think that only exercises involving serious effort get real results, while the opposite is true: if one exercises too seriously, the pressure of one's own expectations can cause tension. Laughter doesn't mean that good exercise principles are being ignored.

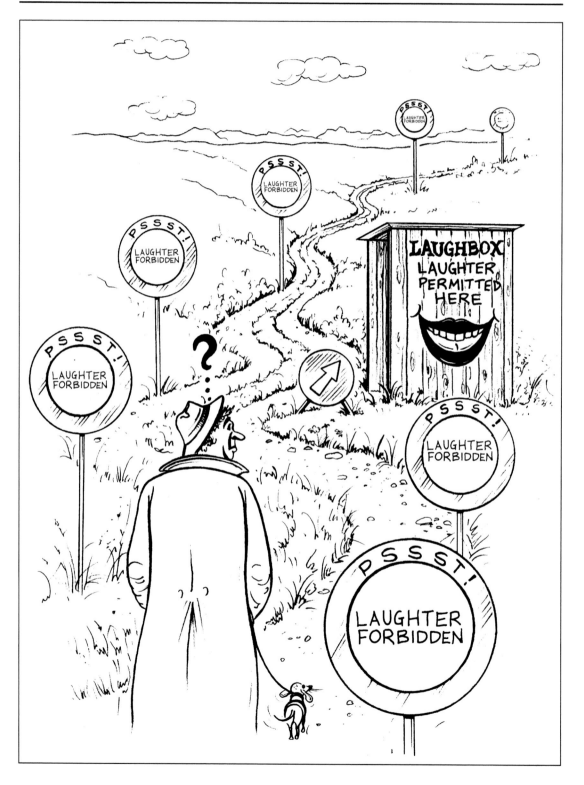

7 Our Daily Routine as Fitness Training

Throughout the day, we have golden opportunities to improve our fitness. If we make the most of these opportunities, we should not be tense and exhausted by evening, but flexible in thought, relaxed in breathing, and well-aligned. Throughout the day, tension builds up in the back, in the shoulders, and in our breathing. In the evening, we try to relax again; but as long as we need relaxation exercises and techniques to do so, it shows that we are constantly becoming tense. Our goal is to reduce our reliance on relaxation techniques, and instead relax with every movement we make.

This is not necessarily easy. At first it may seem strange to work in a relaxed manner, as many of us expect to be tense (especially in our breathing patterns) when we have a lot of work. Many people feel that they have achieved more if they are tired after work. Exhaustion gives us a certain satisfaction, or we may think that our colleagues have more respect for our work if we're exhausted and run-down by the end of the day. If we work in a relaxed fashion, breathing deeply and with a relaxed face and shoulders, our colleagues might suspect us of laziness! However, with time one realizes that the opposite is true. The more relaxed we are, the better our work will be—in both quality and quantity. But the most important thing is that we will be healthier if we work in this way.

Our perceptions depend on our definition of relaxation. Let's not confuse relaxation with slackness or sluggishness. Relaxation means that we are free of superfluous activity in mind and body. Relaxation means the road is cleared for the essential, and we are rid of "tension flab."

Here is a concrete example: while I am writing these lines, two of my children are playing at my desk with anatomical models. My daughter is sitting on my knees. It might become difficult to continue writing, but luckily my "tension monitor" is turned on. As soon as I start to block my breathing even a little, to tense my shoulders or jaw, the monitor will send a message. This helps me to use imagery like "muscles melting" (imagine vanilla ice cream) or "relaxed diaphragm" (like a silk cloth) to relax the areas concerned.

I have discovered again and again that it is far easier to avoid tension from building up than to relax existing cramps and tension. As I continue to breathe deeply and my shoulders are melting, I can nevertheless continue to concentrate wonderfully, even though my chair has just been pushed to the side and I have to adjust my hands to be able to continue typing. In a way, I am doing movement training. The children feel my calm and play peacefully next to me. At this point my son starts to take apart a model of the heart on my desk, and it becomes quite difficult for me to continue breathing calmly (to feel relaxed abdominal breathing and also to melt the shoulders), as I am going to have to take the model away from him. I do take it away; he accepts it, and continues to play. If I had caught my breath and used a tight, tense voice, he might have reacted differently. I am not saying that there aren't moments when one has to interfere clearly and decisively, but very often parents react aggressively because they are tense or exhausted (which is understandable). In the meantime, the liver model has become a hat and a penguin is playing on the stomach model.

The first step toward working in a relaxed way may therefore be to answer the following: are we trying to satisfy society's expectations (regarding the image of a diligent worker), or are we living up to our own image of how we should feel when we have done a good job (exhausted)? The second step is to find out which movements start to make us feel tense. After relaxing fully, when do we start to feel ourselves tensing up again? Where in our body do we tend to become tense? In the shoulders? The neck? In our back? In the jaw? The tongue? The feet? In the belly? The lips? In our breathing? To discover the answer, we have to keep listening to our body. I think that this ability to catch oneself becoming tense is as important as the relaxation exercise itself.

Becoming loose over time requires practice—like almost everything else in life. A child falls down a hundred times before he or she has learned to walk. Only if you are prepared to fail at something at first, can you learn anything. Many people are nevertheless surprised if an exercise or experiment in relaxation or movement doesn't succeed right away.

Our society orients itself more and more toward the immediate satisfaction of desires. But couldn't it be that the good things in life, including a healthy body, are reserved for those who persevere, don't give up, and are willing to start anew again and again?

Inner and outer awareness

1. Grasp an object with your right hand, pick it up and put it down somewhere else. Concentrate on the goal of fulfilling this task. The focus here is on *doing*.

2. Massage the fingertips of your right hand with your left hand. Shake your arm and allow your muscles to be very soft and jelly-like.

3. Again, grasp the same object with your right hand. Concentrate on how this movement feels, and not on the fulfilling of the task. The focus here is on *feeling*.

4. Now try to combine the two aspects. Grasp the object with the goal of moving it and at the same time feel what you are doing. Thus a balance between the doing and sensing part of the nervous system develops. One reason why work can make us so tired and tense is that we focus entirely on the doing—reaching the goal of getting the job done—while hardly feeling ourselves completing the task.

5. Try to apply this in daily life. If you feel that work makes you tired, begin sensing your body while you are working. Your movements will become more precise and you will begin to relax. Do not be concerned with feeling a bit out of place doing this; it is just a new way of doing things. With practice, you will get better at sensing your movements and relaxing while you are busy *doing*.

Waking up the body

At every moment in our lives we have the opportunity for a new beginning. It is never too late to try out something new. You really only start to age once you don't dare to try out new things. If something doesn't work out, don't despair, but rather think: "that wasn't successful; I'll try out something else or try it another way." Every morning is a chance for a fresh start. Even if yesterday didn't turn out the way you wanted it to, you can start the new day with a fresh focus. Have a clear image of how you want to feel in your body throughout the day. Make a wish list for how you would like to feel. This only takes a few

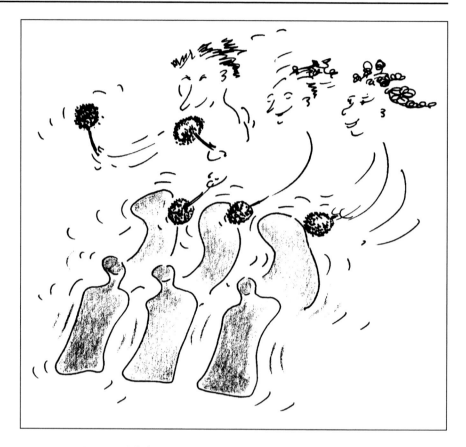

moments. Your wish list can include calm, deep breathing, relaxed muscles, fluid movements, and effortless good posture.

Get into the swing by tapping

Tapping your body in the morning is an excellent way to wake up your body to the new day. You'll use the hands to get the circulation going, wake up the joints and muscles, and get the nervous system alert and ready for the day.

There are different ways of using the hands for tapping. Hold them in loose fists, tap with your fingertips, or with a lightly spread hand.

1. First, gently tap the center of your body, the area around your navel. Feel the tapping waking up your organs.

2. Tap on your breastbone. Feel the heart and lungs waking up through the vibration caused by your hands. Tap from center outward, following the breastbone and the collarbones.

3. Tap along the inside of your arm from the fingertips to the front side of the shoulders and back again. Feel the tapping waking up the muscles, bones, and joints of the arm. Imagine that each cell in your arm is loosened, relaxed, and refreshed.

4. Tap the back of your arm from the side of the neck to the fingertips and back again. Feel the tapping waking up the muscles, bones and joints of your arm.

5. Tap the underside of the arm from the armpit area to the fingertips and back again. Feel the tapping waking up the muscles, bones, and joints of the arm.

6. Compare the feeling between your two arms, before doing the exercise with the other arm. You may notice that the arm and shoulder are more relaxed, the arm feels longer, and its movements more fluid.

7. Now tap the other arm.

8. Now gently tap your head and imagine that the head consists of many bones and joints that are joined in an elastic fashion; the head can be flexible. Also feel the lightness of the bones of the skull.

   You should only attempt the following if you can touch your legs without too much difficulty:

9. Tap the inside of the leg, from the inside edge of the foot to the front of the pelvis.

10. Tap from the front of the leg to the hip joint.

11. Tap from the outside of the foot to the back of the pelvis.

12. Tap on the back of the legs from the heels to the sit bones.

Tapping with Franklin balls is a variation on the exercise above. Use two Franklin balls to tap the body as described above.

A day without friction

Concentrate on your joints and visualize the synovial fluid. Synovia is the fluid that covers the cartilage of your joints, creating a very slippery, friction-free surface for movement. To start a day in which all goes smoothly, at least from the point of view of your joints, concentrate and activate your synovial fluid. Move your right arm in any way that feels comfortable to you and imagine that your movement is stimulating the joints in the arm to produce more synovia. Let the movement reach the shoulder and every bone of your hand and fingers as well. After doing this for a minute or two, rest your arm at your side. You will notice that the muscles have relaxed, and that the shoulder is lower on that side of the body.

Repeat the movement with the other arm and then with each and every joint in your body: the hip joints, knees, feet, spine, neck, and head. Do this gently and imagine that your movements are stimulating the production of synovial fluid.

The portable fitness studio

The Thera-Band ® is a wide elastic rubber band that I like using for exercises. This band is light and easy to transport and fits in any bag. You can use it to train anywhere and anytime, at home, in the office, or on vacation. There are different band strengths; for the following exercise, I recommend a band of medium strength (green or blue). If you don't have such a band, you can also use a bath towel for some of the following exercises.

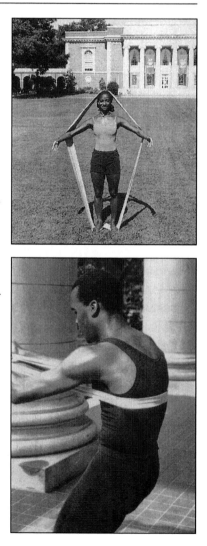

An elastic back in the morning

Standing up, hold the Thera-Band with both hands behind your back. Now bend your spine and let your back rest into the band like a hammock. To do this, move your belly button back and round your spine. Then bring the middle spine forward again. Repeat the movement, let the back push into the band and move the band back and forth—or better yet, wiggle your back into the band as if you wanted to find a comfortable position. Also practice pushing your ribcage sideways against the band. This exercise stretches and tones the back muscles, loosens the ribcage, and thus deepens the breathing. Take the band away and feel how relaxed your back feels, and how freely you can breathe. You may also notice that the spine feels more erect.

Well-oiled shoulders

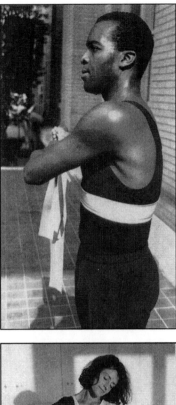

1. For the following exercise, use a long Thera-Band (three to four yards, depending on your body size).

2. Stand with the right foot on both ends of the band. Put the loop of the band over the right shoulder. The loop should stretch neither too tightly nor too loosely over your shoulder.

3. Circle the shoulder within the loop and imagine that the shoulder is well-oiled and lubricated.

4. Bend your head gently to the left. Move your head slowly in different directions. Do not attempt any position that feels uncomfortable. The focus of this exercise is to notice how just a slight change of your head position stretches different muscle groups. Embark on a short and very gentle stretching journey of discovery, and imagine the muscles elongating like chewing gum.

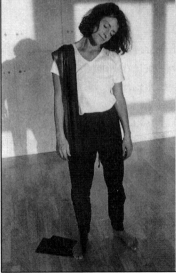

5. Lift your shoulders with the band in the direction of the right ear. Lower them very slowly. Feel the muscles melt like butter.

6. Let go of the band, remove it from your shoulders, and compare the feeling between the "oiled" shoulder and the other shoulder. Then repeat the exercise with the left shoulder.

Getting used to standing

Our feet carry us throughout our lives. We demand a lot of them, but give very little attention to their health. They live in leathery dungeons called shoes from childhood onward, tightly packed, with little air or room for movement. No wonder many people complain about foot pain. But learning just a little about how our feet function is more exciting than a detective novel!

Changeable like a chameleon, the foot takes on a lot of different tasks. To be able to carry so much weight, it is built like a three-dimensional dome. Tensed like a bow, this dome is stable and flexible at the same time. The arch of the foot, with its many ligaments, functions like the string of a bow to store and release energy. The vault of the foot is like the curved body of the bow, and the foot is literally charged with springy energy for every step.

The foot needs to function as a stable foundation, and yet it can also catapult the body forward

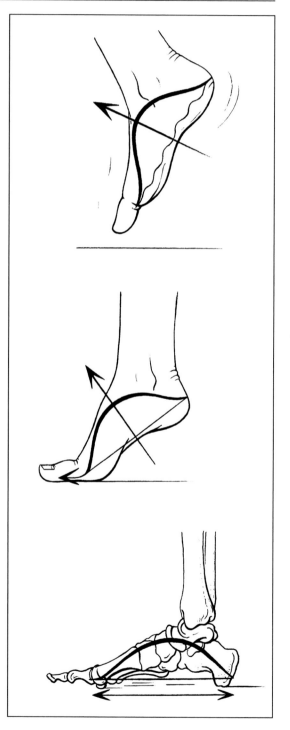

like a lever. It can be flexible or more rigid, depending on what is required at the moment, to lift us from stair to stair or to adapt to the ground. The front part of the foot can even move in the opposite direction to the back part. This trick has saved many a ligament from being overstretched. The back part of the foot can stay upright, even though the front might be tilted to the side by a rock or uneven ground. With its twenty-six bones and more than thirty joints, the foot adapts to every terrain and parries the hardest shocks using the motto "all for one, and one for all." To keep this complex system going, our feet must be utilized fully, all joints and muscles activated regularly. Ideally, our feet should be used as actively as our hands.

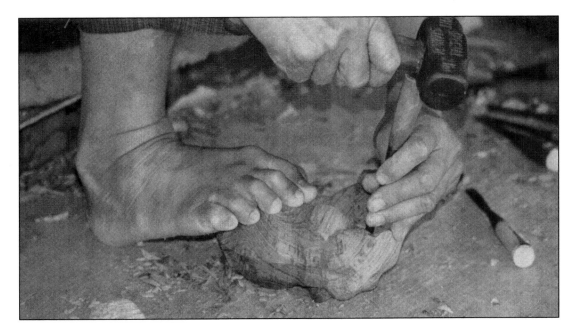

The foot spends most of its life in a shoe and with time it loses the ability to perform its many skills. This has consequences for the whole body. Our circulation is compromised, joints become stiff, muscles become weak, and ligaments thin out. Posture and coordination—and most importantly balance—are closely connected with the state of the feet. Many injuries could be avoided if our sense of balance were exercised regularly.

Before we start exercising, I would like to point to the photograph on the following page. It is of an older woman who spends her day in a boat at the water market in Thailand. She has developed a wonderful sense of balanced posture through her daily confrontation with the demands on her sense of balance. Her whole body is constantly challenged by maneuvering the boat on water amid a myriad of other boats.

To support the body means to challenge it. In the photograph below, we see an illuminating comparison: in the front of the boat, the tourist, and in the back, the local Thai woman steering the boat; in the front a slouched back, and in the back a long, lifted spine. The state of our spine is our choice, and we do not need a boat in order to create better balance and alignment: a simple set of Franklin balls will do.

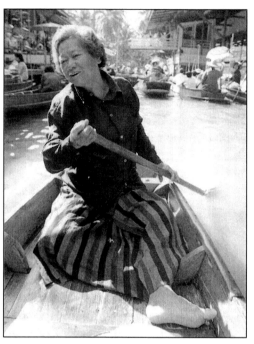

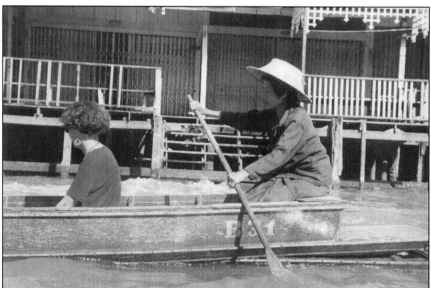

Standing on Franklin balls

The following exercises are more effective than a cup of strong coffee in driving away fatigue. Even though they look easy, they have to be performed with care. Our feet need time to adapt to these new demands. The strength of the feet and a sense of balance have to be built up gradually and progressively.

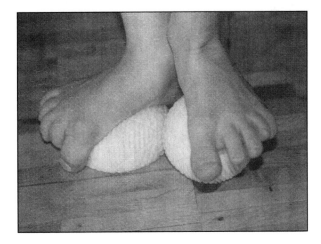

1. Start with one foot on a ball, and keep the other on the ground. Keep the heel on the ground and move the front of the foot across the ball to the left and back to the right. Move the foot until the side touches the ground, then go to the other side. Do this vigorously for about a minute.

2. Now put the ball of the same foot on the ground and the heel on the ball. Press on the ball with your heel. Move the heel back and forth on the ball, keeping the ball of the foot on the floor.

3. Put the arch of the foot on the ball, with the middle of the foot resting on the ball. Push down onto the ball by shifting your weight forward, then rock back again. As you rock forward, feel your weight on the ball, not merely the pressure from the strength of your leg. Repeat this rocking and ball-squashing action at least twenty times.

4. Step off the ball and compare your two feet on the flat ground. You may notice many things at this point: the foot feels flatter, and more spread out; the arch feels higher; the whole side of the body where your foot was working out is more relaxed. Maybe you can also feel a difference in your shoulders. If you balance on the workout side, you will feel more stable as well. You will notice this especially if you close your eyes and try balancing on first one, then the other, foot.

The following exercise builds up strength and flexibility in the feet and legs, strengthens the bones and muscles, and improves balance and posture. It is the next phase of ball balancing, and involves standing on both balls at the same time. For this I recommend holding onto something stable. You may also do the exercise with a partner, facing and holding onto each other.

1. Step onto one ball, then the other.

2. See if you can gently bounce on the balls, relaxing your shoulders. Breathe deeply.

3. If you can, let go of your partner for a moment.

4. Bend and stretch your legs on the balls.

5. If you are able to let go of your partner, practice lifting and lowering your shoulders while standing on the balls.

6. For a bit of a calf stretch, just place the balls of the feet on the (Franklin) balls while the heels touch the floor.

7. Also try the opposite: put the balls under the heels while the toes touch the floor. Step off the balls and notice your posture. Standing is effortless, the shoulders are relaxed, and you feel calm and grounded.

Incidentally, kids love this game and it is interesting to watch how they balance on their feet.

Sitting for strength and flexibility

In the Western world, millions of people spend their day flattening their buttocks that contain the strongest muscle in the body, the *gluteus maximus*. This muscle is not being exercised; instead it starts to adapt to the width of the increasingly comfortable seat. In the United States, the seats of one old stadium had to be replaced; in the past, spectators needed only half the surface area for their buttocks! Let us courageously stand (or sit) against this worldwide trend. The following exercises are not only advantageous for the gluteal muscles, abdominal muscles and a good sitting posture, but they also activate the pelvic floor.

Exercising on a chair

1. Sitting down, locate your sit bones, which can be found at the bottom of the pelvis. Put your hands under your buttocks. You will probably find the pressure of the two bones unpleasantly compressing your fingers. Take your hands away again and feel whether the weight of your body is equally distributed on both of these bones.

2. Now press the right sit bone into the chair seat with more effort

than the left one. Imagine that it is pressing into a piece of clay (the chair) and making an indentation. Release the right sit bone and press the left sit bone into the chair, using the same image. Which one is easier to press into the chair? If you notice a difference, it is a sign of muscular imbalance. Our goal is to have balanced muscle strength in the pelvic floor, for it will greatly benefit your lower back and posture in general.

3. Try to walk on the chair with your sit bones. This will work best if the chair is level and not too soft. Imagine that this is the same action as walking on two feet. One of the sit bones pushes off the chair, while the other stretches forward (see illustration). Also try moving backward. The reason you can do this is that in humans, walking is very much driven by a twisting action of the spine, and not by the legs.

4. Lift the right buttock slightly off the chair, so that you are only balanced on the left sit bone. Now swing the right buttock back and forth a few times. Imagine you're dusting off the chair with

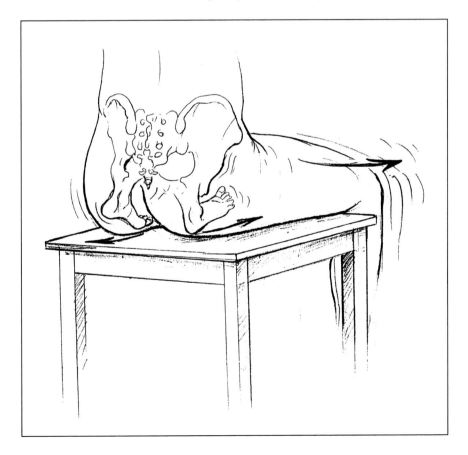

your sit bones as though they are little brushes. Compare the feeling in the lower back muscles before performing the same action on the left side. Slightly lift the left side of the pelvis off the seat so that you are only "standing" on the right sit bone. Swing the left buttock a few times back and forth, again imagining the sit bone as a brush that is sweeping the surface of the chair.

5. Try to pull the sit bones together as if they were being magnetically attracted, and then release them again. Imagine a ball of wool between the sit bones. Squeeze the ball with your sit bones and then let go if it again. Repeat the action three times.

6. Take a break from "sit bone gymnastics" with a breathing exercise. Imagine you can breathe into the area between the sit bones. Can you feel them drawing just slightly apart while inhaling, and drawing together again when you are exhaling? You can use each breath to exercise the pelvic floor.

And finally, two playful advanced exercises with Franklin balls:

1. Put two Franklin balls under the sit bones and try to balance on them. If it feels unpleasant, you can put a towel on top of the balls. Balance on the balls for at least two minutes. Move and squirm on the balls as if you were a child anxiously waiting for recess.

2. How does your pelvis feel after you have taken away the balls? You may notice that your sitting posture is more upright and that there is more firmness in your abdominal muscles.

1. Can you get up from the chair and allow your arms and shoulders to be relaxed and calm?

2. Imagine that your sit bones are pushing you forward while standing up, as if there was a magic carpet between them. Gently glide down again with this carpet.

3. To stand up, imagine a thread attached to the pubic bone pulling you up and continuing to pull you forward until you're walking around the room.

4. When you sit down, imagine the sit bones as a rocket booster cushioning your descent. Make sure your pelvis lands softly on the chair: no plunking down, for which your lower back is grateful.

5. Imagine pleasant, warm water running down your back when you stand up. When you sit down, feel sand trickling down your knees.

We can learn a great deal about good posture from watching children. Children are expert at sitting down, standing up, and lifting objects. Look at the wonderfully balanced posture of the two-year-old in the photograph.

Supported by the coccyx and the pelvic floor, a clear elongation of the spine can be seen: a stance with legs wide apart, feet and knees pointing forward, and the hip joints kept low in order to be able to relieve the back with the gluteal muscles. A two-year-old back health expert!

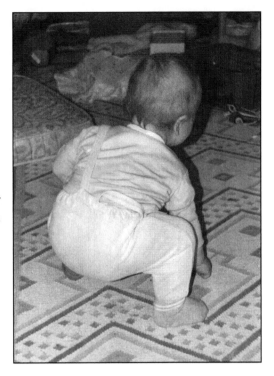

The body-friendly office

My recommendations for office fitness may not correspond to the norm. For instance, I do not suggest more expensive chairs, but simpler ones instead. While leading workshops, I am often asked which chair I would recommend. My response is a flat wooden chair, perhaps with a cushion on top. A chair that is too comfortable will tempt us into a slouched sitting posture. Choose a chair that encourages you to get up and move about from time to time. Put a lot of spice and variation into your sitting routine: sit on two Franklin balls, sometimes even on the floor (if circumstances permit), or work (read a report) while walking or standing. Frequently used envelopes and stamps should not necessarily be within easy reaching distance, but should make you stretch your arms, get up from your chair, or even to take a little walk. Hardly the concept for an efficient office? Not true. If your body gets more movement, you feel healthier and work with increased concentration and stamina.

Here is a series of exercises for the office that you can do without attracting too much attention. A colleague or two may even be tempted to try some of the exercises.

Shoulder relaxation with Franklin balls and gentle stretching

1. While standing up, place your Franklin balls in your armpits for a few moments. Rhythmically press against and release the balls about five times. Now take the balls away and feel your shoulders. Have they dropped a bit? That is a sign of relaxation.

2. Put the balls back under the armpits. Lift your shoulders and lower them again with the balls under your armpits. As the shoulders lower, imagine them melting down over the balls. I like to image them as scoops of ice cream, and my shoulders as warm chocolate sauce melting over the ice cream. (If you're not an ice cream person, simply imagine your shoulder blades as heavy sacks of flour or sugar). Their weight helps to lengthen the shoulder muscles as the shoulders lower. Remove the balls and notice your shoulders, neck, and spine. The shoulders may feel as if they have dropped, and the muscles and the spine may feel lengthened.

3. Take the balls away and put your right hand on your left shoulder. Tilt your head carefully to the right until you feel a slight stretching of your neck muscles. Breathe calmly and imagine your shoulders are like melting butter (or ice cream, as above). Lift your head slowly into an upright position again. Repeat the lowering and lifting of the head with your hand on your shoulder three more times, always using an image that works for you to enhance the relaxation of the muscles. Then take your right hand off your left shoulder and compare the state of your right and left shoulders. You may notice that the left shoulder has dropped once again.

4. Now put your left hand on your right shoulder and bend your head carefully to the left until you feel a slight stretching of your neck muscles. Breathe as calmly as possible. Imagine that your shoulders are melting like butter. Lift your head slowly into an upright position again. Repeat the action three times. Notice the changes in your shoulder. You are mastering the art of tension relief. This will clear your head and make you feel calmer and in control. Stretch your arms forward with a rounded back. Now try to lift your shoulders a little and push them down again. Imagine your shoulder blades sliding smoothly on your rib cage.

5. Stand upright, shake your arms a bit and enjoy your new shoulders!

Eye relaxation in the office

Our eyes are located in conical pyramid-shaped eye sockets and are surrounded by muscles and a padding of fat. There is a clear liquid in the inner part of the eye. It is especially important to relax the eyes regularly if you spend a lot of time working at a computer screen. Wash your hands before the next exercise, even if your hands are clean, as the purpose 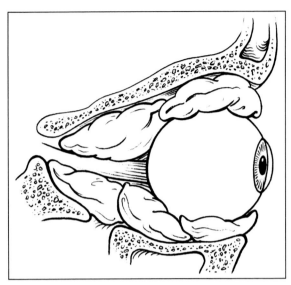 of the exercise is to give the eyes a feeling of freshness.

1. Circle the edges of your eye sockets with your fingertips. Be aware that the eye sockets are made up of many different bones; the eyes are encased in a rigid capsule but surrounded by tiny flexible bones. Under the eye is the upper jaw bone, toward the outside of the eye is the temporal bone, and above the eye is the frontal bone. The inner side of the eye is made up of many different thin-walled nasal bones. This knowledge alone can help to relax one's eyes.

2. Place your (clean) hands on your eyes, comfortably embedded in the eye sockets. Imagine that your eyes are surrounded by silk cushions into which they can sink with a sigh of relaxation.

3. Imagine that your eyes are filling with crystal-clear spring water. Any cloudiness in the eyes disappears.

Fresh air for the cells

Get up and open the window to let some fresh air into the room. Imagine that each cell of your body is being aired out. For those who are especially imaginative, visualize the cell membranes being moved lightly by a breath of air, like a sail fluttering in the wind.

Forest air in the office

If you can't open the window, then you can still imagine that you are sitting in a forest surrounded by the energy of trees and plants. Also imagine the sounds of the forest and the pleasant smell of the plants. Feel how every cell of your body is refreshed by these pleasant surroundings and is encouraged to breathe deeply.

The brain as a sea anemone in the office

You may be surprised to know that it's possible to relax the brain. In this exercise we will relax a brain that might be a bit tense after the stresses of the day. Every part of the body can be relaxed; should the muscles alone have this privilege? The result of relaxation is that one uses only the necessary effort for the task at hand and no more. This will increase concentration and endurance. Our brain and spinal cord float in a liquid called the spinal fluid. This liquid surrounds our valuable brain cells, protecting and nourishing them, and cushioning them from blows. Our brain could be viewed as a kind of commander in chief, urging our body to perform at its full potential, but this organ is also in a permanent bathing spa! Imagine the brain, including the spinal cord, floating like a sea anemone. Look at the illustration on page 42 or think of an aquarium for inspiration.

Zen and the art of vacuum cleaning

Being more aware of your own movements can make boring work more interesting. Instead of wearing yourself out with exhausting housework or physical work of any kind, you can transform it into a game. You may use a vacuum cleaner, as suggested below, or any other household or gardening device to practice body-conscious movement.

As you get out the vacuum cleaner, ask yourself: "can I keep my shoulders loose and breathe calmly as I vacuum?" Even if the answer is "no," continue with the exercise. Imagine your shoulders melting like warm beeswax. Feel the wax melting. Maybe you can even smell its pleasant scent. Observe your rhythmic breathing. If you want to laugh while doing this, even better, as this exercise is not without its comical side.

Now start with the actual work. It doesn't matter how fast you are. While working, place your awareness on your shoulders, and then on your breathing. Perhaps it's difficult for you to think of your shoulders melting as you vacuum, but with time your body will learn to work in a relaxed way without having to think about it. Perhaps you can remember learning to drive, when you had to think carefully about every maneuver. Now it's much easier!

After about three or four minutes, stand quietly. Concentrate on your shoulders again, and imagine them melting like ice cream. Be aware of your breathing. Allow it to be deep and soft. You can imagine that the air you're breathing relaxes your lungs, as if it were massaging them from inside. Repeat the sequence "standing-concentrating/working-concentrating" three times. Afterward ask yourself: "do I feel more relaxed than before?" At this point many people discover that they have actually become more relaxed while working.

A big step toward a healthier lifestyle is discovering that work, any kind of work, can relax the body.

Taking care of the garden and your back

As soon as you pick up your spade, remember that when you dig you shouldn't bend your back; use your legs and hip joints, and lower your center of gravity. This requires a certain elasticity of the pelvic floor, as a lack of flexibility in the hip joints starts here. For many people, proper bending isn't easy, but for this reason it should be practiced more often. Otherwise enormous strain is put on the spine. Children know spontaneously how to dig in the right way. Have a child teach you, and imagine that your own body is just as elastic and flexible.

Breathing into the skull

The skull is not a hard case imprisoning our brain. Let go of this unfavorable image and imagine that you can breathe into the skull and experience it as soft and malleable. See if you notice any movement of the skull when you breathe. This is difficult, so lightly tap the head with your fingertips, with the awareness that the skull consists of many individual bones. Afterwards try to "breathe into the head" again; it will be much easier now.

The subtle movements of the head during inhalation and exhalation can be seen very clearly in a newborn baby. A baby offers the best visual instruction for breathing with the whole body. Imagine the breath in the bones of your skull, and you'll see that it's a great way to prevent headaches.

Walking on feathers

Stand on the landing of a staircase and hold onto the railing. Stand on one leg and let the other leg hang over the edge of the first stair. Swing the leg loosely back and forth as if it were a rope dangling from the hip joint. After two to three minutes, walk around a bit and compare the feeling in the two legs. You will notice that the leg that has been swinging feels very relaxed and free. Repeat the exercise with the other leg. If you do not have a staircase, then you can stand on a raised surface or anything that will lift you off the ground a few inches.

Supportive wind

As you walk, imagine a pleasant wind at just the right temperature pushing you forward. The legs move almost of their own accord. The center of your body is in front of the sacrum. If you imagine that the pushing action comes from behind, against the back of the pelvis (see illustration), then you will achieve a particularly relaxed walk.

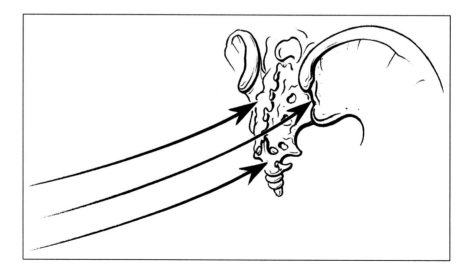

Imagine that threads are attached to the tips of your toes. These threads pull your feet rhythmically forward as you walk.

Disk balloons

Imagine that the disks between the vertebrae are like small balloons that help to lift and lengthen the spine. These small balloons lift the vertebrae from below so that you can sense your spine as a chain of floating segments.

Exercising in line

In addition to all the exercises we have talked about so far, there are, of course, many more daily opportunities for a bit of exercise. Don't get annoyed when you have to wait for a friend, a train, bus, or cab. This may be the chance to perform a bit of mental relaxation or postural awareness. Even a traffic holdup can be turned into an opportunity to loosen your neck and shoulder muscles, to breathe deeply, and replenish your energy.

Letting the first rib float

The first rib forms a circle at the top of the ribcage. If it is compressed and slouching forward, that may cause neck and upper back tension. Imagine the first rib to be free and buoyant, like a circular piece of cork floating on water. If the first rib is elevated and floating, the heart and lungs will be decompressed, and more oxygen will be available to fuel a happy life!

Delight in taking the stairs

Aerobics play a part of everyday fitness activities, too. We can turn every staircase into an aerobics training ground. Let's think of a day in a typical town or city: it's not only wheelchair users who shudder when faced with a flight of stairs. Pedestrians in the subway have long since become used to being transported upward by some remote power source, and thus avoid having to rely on their own two legs. We need escalators and elevators for the handicapped, of course, but the rest of us should make the most of the opportunity to improve our fitness by taking the stairs. When you are confronted with a staircase, do not despair. Instead tell yourself the following: "I will make the most of this! I will exercise my muscles in a balanced fashion. My legs will become more attractive. My heart and lungs will get a nice workout. This is an opportunity for my whole body!" Then, as you walk up the stairs, keep focusing on all the benefits. You will be surprised at how good you feel!

Marionette

Imagine you are a puppet being carried along by thin yet strong threads. The threads are attached to your knees, pulling them up. Another thread is attached to your head and takes care of the lifting and lengthening of your spine. Further threads are attached to your elbows to take the weight off your arms. When you go down the stairs, the same threads make sure that your legs are lowered slowly and elegantly. The foot is gently placed onto each step. The spine stays upright, and you simply float down the stairs.

The ball

Imagine that you are bouncing like a ball from stair to stair. Even the stairs themselves are rubbery and resilient, as if they were pushing you upward like the surface of a trampoline. You alone can choose to adapt to your environment. Why not therefore transform it into something supportive for your body?

Restful sleep

Sleep is our chance to replenish our minds and bodies. Not just the quantity, but the quality of sleep is important. Mental and physical preparation for sleep is just as important as a good bed. Falling into bed exhausted is not a good start for a restful night's sleep. We have read advice telling us that eating a large meal before going to bed will affect our sleep. However, we should not go to bed hungry. The same is true of mental nourishment. What we read just before going to sleep is important; it can continue to affect our entire organism throughout the night. Ideally we should read something positive and uplifting, or literature with a positive message. Detective novels and horror stories are not conducive to a good night's sleep, as their subject matter can weave itself into our dreams and disturb our sleep. Obviously the same holds true for watching television. If you must watch before sleep, choose images that you want to go to bed with.

Constructive sleep

The evening is an ideal time for the Constructive Rest Position (see page 33). It is highly recommended that you take at least fifteen minutes for this. It's worth it, as you'll sleep more deeply and feel more rested and fresher the next day. Here are some ideas to help you fall asleep, and then to sleep deeply:

1. Lie on the floor (or on a mat) in the CRP, relax your whole body, and imagine that all the parts of your body are sinking into the floor like heavy sacks of flour.

2. Imagine that your back is resting and sinking into warm, soft clay.

3. Let your back spread out on the ground like melting butter.

4. Hang your legs over an imaginary clothes hanger.

    Or

5. Choose one of the many CRP images described in this book.

Embracing mother earth

Lie down on your stomach on soft padding. You may want to place a pillow under your hip joints and belly. In this position you can clearly feel your breathing. Your stomach pushes against the floor when you inhale, and relaxes when you exhale. Feel the pressure of your body against the floor and imagine that you are lying on a large sphere. It is almost as if you were embracing the earth. Imagine that the earth itself is breathing below you. After a few minutes, try to grasp the earth beneath you with your hands and your whole body. In this way, you will activate the muscles in the front of your body, helping you to relax your back muscles once you stand up again.

Franklin balls: a flexibility exercise for the evening

Exercises with Franklin balls are very suitable for the evening because they help you fall asleep with a loose and relaxed body. The balls support the subtle coordination of the muscles, creating joint-saving movements. We will use images to increase the effect of the balls.

The balls should lie between the floor and the body, enabling a new kind of muscle initiation with a relaxing effect on the joints and muscles. When we work with the balls in a lying position, we don't have to worry about our posture and can concentrate completely on our movements. The benefits of exercising with balls follow:

1. Physical massage of the muscles and loosening of tension take place in the connective tissues, both of which will improve flexibility. Circulation is improved within the muscles.

2. Our joints will be lubricated. Production of synovial fluid is increased. The ball compresses the vessels and immediately lets them expand to their full size. This stretching and widening of the vessels allows for a better detoxification of the tissues.

3. The micro-movements made while rolling on the balls eliminate unfavorable posture patterns and help to build new ones.

4. Breathing is crucial to the success of rolling exercises with the balls. The balls are like mobile sensory devices that show us

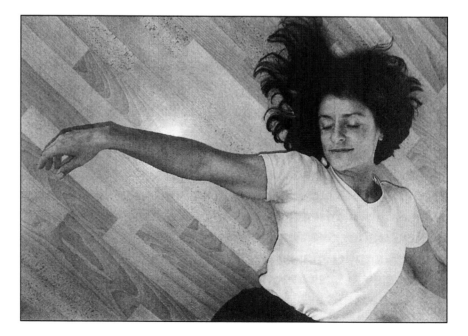

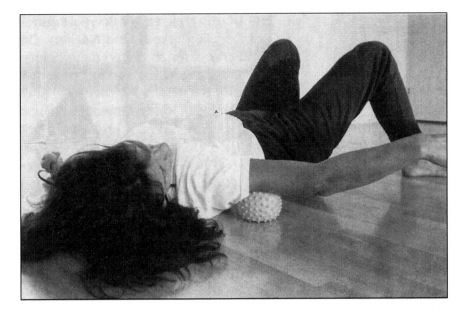

the exact state of tension in our muscles. Our breath can be directed toward a tense muscle, entering the muscle and loosening it in the process. During exhalation, we allow all tension to flow out of our body.

The more complete our breathing, the more tension will be eliminated. As soon as we discover a sore spot, we have a tendency to hold our breath. But with time we notice that if we breathe into the center of the pain, it starts to dissolve. If one loosens tension somewhere in the body, the entire body reacts with relaxation. We are only as relaxed as the most tense part of our body.

The most important points to remember when rolling on the Franklin balls are as follows:

1. Never roll the balls over an injury or a slipped disk.

2. Move slowly and continuously. Rolling on the balls should resemble a very slow dance. The most effective movement is slow and flowing.

3. Breathe as freely as possible; sigh from time to time, or yawn whenever you feel like it.

4. Remove the balls if you experience pain, dizziness or a tingling in the arms or legs. This is simply due to pressure on an artery, and will be relieved as soon as you remove the balls.

Loosening the pelvis and lower back

Lie down on your back and place the balls under your buttocks. Start to move your pelvis slowly. Try to vary your movements as much as possible. Move the pelvis sideways, back and forth, and rotate it in imaginative ways.

Creating flexible shoulders

1. Lie down on your back and place a ball under your right upper arm.

2. Move the upper arm in several different ways.

3. Try to initiate your movements from the shoulder blade.

4. Compare the feeling in both shoulders before doing the exercise with the left arm.

Relaxing the *latissimus dorsi* and pectoral muscle

1. Lie down on your back and place two balls under the upper part of your back and one ball under your head.

2. Lift your arms straight up in the air.

3. Lower your arms to the ground. During this exercise remember to relax your spine; imagine it sinking into the floor.

4. Repeat this sequence three times. Then take the balls away and see how your back feels.

In the following exercise we will try to create space for movement between the back of the head and the neck. We often move as if these two parts of the body were glued together, but for turning and twisting movements, and also for the entire spine, it is very important to loosen the neck muscles. Even in those of us with a slouched upper body, postural reflexes lift the head so that our eyes look up and forward. The result is permanently shortened neck muscles. That's why this exercise should be done with the utmost awareness. At the slightest sign of dizziness, you should take the ball away and rest until the dizziness has passed.

1. Lie down on your back and place a ball under your head. The surface should be such that the ball doesn't roll or slip away.

2. The mat that you are lying on should be thick enough to prevent the cervical spine from becoming overly flexed.

3. Slowly turn your head sideways on the ball; your line of vision will change as you look more and more to the side. This movement should be done with as much flow as possible.

4. Turn the head only as far as feels pleasant, and turn it back again slowly.

5. Now do the same movement on the other side. Make note of any differences between your left and right sides.

6. Repeat the movement as often as you like.

7. Do your neck and back feel different? Focus on the new feeling.

Bibliography and references

Achterberg, J. *Imagery in Healing*. Boston and London: Shambhala Publications, 1985.

Alexander, A. *Eutonie*. München, Germany: Kösel Verlag, 1976.

Bäumlein-Schurter, M. *Übungen zur Konzentration*. Zürich: Origo-Verlag, 1966.

Blakeslee, S. "Animals That Are Peerless Athletes." *Science Times of The New York Times*, 1 June 1993.

———. "Seeing and Imagining: Clues to the Workings of the Mind's Eye." *Science Times of The New York Times*, 31 August 1993.

Chopra, D. *Quantum Healing*. New York: Bantam Books, 1990.

Clark, B. "Body Proportion Needs Depth—Front to Back." Champaign, IL: Published by the author, 1975.

———. "How to Live in Your Axis—Your Vertical Line". Port Washington, NY: Published by the author, 1968.

———. "Let's Enjoy Sitting—Standing—Walking." Port Washington, NY: Published by the author, 1963

Clouser, J. "The Grand Plié: Some Physiological and Ethical Considerations." *Impulse*. Champaign, IL: Human Kinetics (1994) 83–86.

Cohen, B. *Sensing, Feeling, and Action: The Experiential Anatomy of Body–Mind Centering*. Northampton, MA: Contact Editions, 1980.

———. "The Alphabet of Movement." *Contact Quarterly*, 28 January 1988.

Dart, R.A. "Voluntary Musculature in the Human Body: The Double Spiral Arrangement." *The British Journal of Physical Medicine*. London: Butterworth (1950) 265–268.

Dowd, I. *Taking Root to Fly*. Northampton, MA: Contact Editions, 1990.

Durkheim. *Hara, the Vital Center of Man*. London: Allen and Unwin, 1992.

Epstein, G., M.D. *Healing Visualizations*. New York: Bantam Books, 1989.

Feldenkrais, M. *Awareness Through Movement*. New York: Harper Collins, 1972.

Feuerstein, G. *The Shambhala Guide to Yoga*. Boston and London: Shambhala Publications, 1996.

Flanagan, O. *The Science of Mind*. Cambridge, MA: MIT Press, 1991.

Franklin, E. *Dance Imagery for Technique and Performance*. Champaign, IL: Human Kinetics, 1996.

———. *Dynamic Alignment through Imagery*. Champaign, IL: Human Kinetics, 1996.

———. *Pelvic Power: Mind/Body Exercises for Strength, Flexibility, Posture, and Balance for Men and Women*. Hightstown, NJ: Princeton Book Co., Publishers, 2003.

———. *Relax your Neck, Liberate your Shoulders: The Ultimate Exercise Program for Tension Relief*. Hightstown, NJ: Princeton Book Co. Publishers, 2001.

Ghose, A. *Integral Yoga: Sri Aurobindo's Teaching and Method of Practice*. Twin Lakes, WI: Lotus Press, 1997.

Hotz, A., and J. Weineck. *Optimales Bewegungslernen*. Erlangen, Germany: Perimed, 1983.

Jacobsen, E. "Electrical Measurements of Neuromuscular States During Mental Activities: Imagination of Movement Involving Skeletal Muscle." *American Journal of Physiology* (1929) 91:597–608.

Jones, S., R. Martin, and D. Pilbeam, Eds. *Cambridge Encyclopedia of Human Evolution*. Cambridge: Cambridge University Press, 1992.

Juhan, D. *Job's Body*. Barrytown, NY: Station Hill Press, 1987.

Keeleman, C.S. *Emotional Anatomy*. Berkeley, CA: Center Press, 1985.

Kendal, P. *Muscle Testing and Function*. Baltimore, MD: Williams and Wilkins, 1983.

Klein–Vogelbach, S. *Funktionelle Bewegungslehre*. Berlin: Springer, 1997.

Kükelhaus. *Hören und Sehen in Tätigkeit*. Zug, Switzerland: Klett und Balmer, 1978.

———. *Unmenschliche Architektur*. Köln, Germany: Gaia Verlag, 1988.

Lee, D. *The Pelvic Girdle, An Approach to the Examination and Treatment of the Lumbo–Pelvic–Hip Region*. London: Churchill Livingstone, 2000.

Masunaga, S. *Zen Imagery Exercises*. Tokyo: Japan Publications, 1987.

Maxwell, M. *Human Evolution*. Sidney, Australia: Croom Helm, 1984.

Merlau–Ponty, M. *Phenomenology of Perception*. London: Routledge, 1962.

Mookerjee, A. *Kundalini: The Arousal of Inner Energy*. Rochester, VT: Destiny Books, 1982.

Norkin, C., and P. Levangie. *Joint Structure and Function*. Philadelphia, PA: F.A. Davis, 1992.

Ohashi, W. *Reading the Body*. New York: Penguin Books, 1991.

Olsen, A. *Body Stories: A Guide to Experiential Anatomy*. Barrytown, NY: Station Hill Press, 1991.

Park, G. *The Art of Changing*. Bath, England: Ashgrove Press, 1989.

Pascal, E. *Jung to Live By*. New York: Warner Books, 1992.

Pierce, A., and R. Pierce. *Expressive Movement*. New York: DaCapo Press, div. of Perseus, 2002.

Porterfield, J., and C. DeRosa. *Mechanical Lower Back Pain: Perspectives in Functional Anatomy*. Philadelphia, PA: Saunders and Co., 1991.

Radin, E., et al. *Practical Biomechanics for the Orthopedic Surgeon*. New York: Churchill Livingstone, 1992.

Rolfingsmeier, T. "Using Biofeedback to Address Male Incontinence." *Advance for Physical Assistants and PT Assistants* (2003) 14:14.

Rolland, J. *Inside Motion: An Ideokinetic Basis for Movement Education*. Urbana, IL: Rolland String Research Associates, 1984.

Rossi, E. *The Psychobiology of Mind–Body Healing: New Concepts of Therapeutic Hypnosis*. New York: W. W. Norton & Company, 1986.

Samuels, M., and N. Samuels. *Seeing with the Mind's Eye*. New York: Random House, 1975.

Sherrington, C. *Man on his Nature*. New York: Mentor Books, 1964.

Sweigard, L. Reprint of "The Dancer and His Posture" in *Annual of Contemporary Dance. Impulse*. San Francisco (1961) 3.

———. *Human Movement Potential: Its Ideokinetic Facilitation*. New York: Dodd, Mead and Company, 1978.

Todd, M. *Early Writings, 1920-1934*. Reprint. New York: Dance Horizons.

———. *The Hidden You*. Reprint. New York: Dance Horizons, 1953.

———. *The Thinking Body*. 1937. Reprint. New York: Dance Horizons, 1972.

Verin, L. "The Teaching of Moshe Feldenkrais." In *Your Body Works*. G. Kogan, ed. Berkeley, CA: And/Or Press (1980) 83-86.

Werner, H., ed. *The Body Percept*. New York: Random House, 1965.

White, R. "Visual Thinking in the Ice Age." *Scientific American* (1989) 261: 1, 74.

Index

Appendix: Franklin Method Resources

other books by Eric Franklin

Relax Your Neck, Liberate Your Shoulders: The Ultimate Exercise Program for Tension Relief
and
*Pelvic Power: Mind/body Exercises for Strength, Flexibility, Posture,
and Balance for Men and Women*

Princeton Book Company, Publishers, Hightstown, NJ, USA

Conditioning for Dance, Breakdance, Dance Imagery for Technique and Performance,
and *Dynamic Alignment Through Imagery*

Human Kinetics, Champaign, IL, USA

workshops

Workshops and teacher trainings, open to everybody, are regularly offered on the topics
covered in this book as well as other aspects of movement and therapy.

Visit our web page at: www.franklin-methode.ch

Or contact us at:
Institut für Franklin-Methode, Brunnenstrassse 1, CH–8610 Uster, Switzerland

email: info@franklin-methode.ch

The exercise balls ("Franklin balls") used in exercises in this book can be ordered from
Orthopedic Physical Therapy Products (www.optp.com).